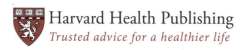

Dear Reader,

It's no secret by now that two in three American adults weigh too much. The question is, why? As it turns out, there isn't one simple answer. We know that genes are part of the picture, but our genes haven't changed much in the past few generations. What has changed dramatically is the world we live in. Today, we're often too pressed for time or too tired to prepare meals at home from scratch. When we dine out or order takeout instead, portions are huge. We've also become a snacking society, and we frequently choose unhealthy snacks and eat them mindlessly. Add in fewer opportunities to be physically active in the normal course of the day, soaring stress levels, and reduced amounts of sleep—all of which can lead to comfort eating—and you have a recipe for weight gain. Certain prescription medications may add to the problem by increasing your hunger. And once you put on extra pounds, your body wants to maintain that new weight, making it hard to reverse course.

That's why it's time to stop blaming yourself and put that mental energy into taking action instead. Weight loss depends less on willpower than "skill power." Overweight and obesity are complex conditions with many different causes and treatment options. There is no one-size-fits-all strategy. However, this isn't the message we hear in the media and online where extreme, unrealistic—and sometimes unhealthy—diet advice runs rampant. Some of this may work for the short term, but it fails in the long run, turning us into a nation of yo-yo dieters, stuck in a lose-regain-repeat cycle.

If simply wanting to lose weight was enough, we'd all be thin. Maybe the approaches you tried in the past just weren't right for you. Maybe you weren't quite ready to change—or confident that you could change. Now's the time to make a fresh start. Throughout this newly revised and updated Special Health Report, you'll discover many different strategies that you can tailor to your own needs and lifestyle to help you reach your goals. For some people, that might mean changes in eating and exercise habits. Others may require medication or possibly surgery. And because knowing what—and how much—to eat can be one of the biggest roadblocks, we've also included seven days' worth of meal suggestions in the Special Section of this report.

In the end, weight loss isn't just about a number on the scale. It's about cultivating a healthy lifestyle, developing positive ways to deal with food, and setting realistic, achievable goals to help you to weather that storm and emerge healthier and more energetic, for the long term.

Sincerely,

Florencia Halperin, M.D.
Medical Editor

Carrie Dennett, M.P.H., R.D.N., L.D.
Nutrition Editor

The editors would like to acknowledge Dr. W. Scott Butsch and nutritionist Karen Ansel, who created the previous version of this report.

Harvard Health Publishing | Harvard Medical School | 4 Blackfan Circle, 4th Floor | Boston, MA 02115

Why is it so hard to lose weight?

Anyone who has ever been on a diet can tell you that losing weight is hard work—but keeping it off can be even harder. Only about 20% of people who lose weight maintain their losses for longer than a year. However, with the right tools, long-lasting change is possible. Whether you're trying to lose 5 pounds or 50, this Special Health Report will offer practical, achievable advice and tips to help you shed excess weight healthfully while still eating food that is delicious and satisfying. For those who need greater weight reduction, it will also offer information on weight-loss medication and surgery.

But first, it helps to understand why losing weight is so tough. The truth is, weight loss isn't just about eating fewer calories or having more willpower. It's a far more complex interchange of biology, genetics, food choices, and environment.

Biology—whose side is it on?

From an evolutionary perspective, our bodies were designed to store fat for times of famine. This may have been helpful thousands of years ago when we had to hunt and gather our food, but today, when there's often more than enough food to go around, the body's drive to squirrel away fat for lean times is working against us.

In this pursuit for survival, the body is assisted by stubborn hormones such as leptin and ghrelin, which ensure that you won't starve to death, but which can also undermine willpower. If you've ever found it impossible to lose those last 5 or 10 pounds, blame it on these two hormones. The first, leptin, is produced by your fat cells. Like a gas gauge in a car, it tells your brain when you have enough fuel on board. When you lose weight, a low leptin level signals your brain that you are going on empty and need to fill up. The other hormone, ghrelin, is made in your stomach and intestine and works the opposite way. When you haven't eaten for a few hours, *rising* levels let your brain know that it's time to eat again. Ghrelin levels also increase when you lose weight, prompting you to eat more and simultaneously slowing your metabolism—the rate at which your body uses calories.

Even though you may desperately want to shed excess fat, your brain has other plans—namely, hanging on to as much fat as it thinks you require for survival. To this end, it works like a thermostat, constantly monitoring levels of hormones such as leptin that provide feedback on body fat levels. When you eat less and lose weight, your brain jumps in, working to restore equilibrium by sending out hunger signals and—to make matters worse—slowing your metabolism (see "Lessons from 'The Biggest Loser,'" page 3).

The brain's reward system only adds to the challenge by encouraging you to seek out high-fat, high-calorie food—a strategy that used to aid survival in times when food was scarce, but works to our detriment today. While our biology hasn't changed much, our food supply has, especially over the past 40 or so years—a very rapid change in the context of the nearly 200,000 years of human evolution. Today, 58% of the food we eat consists of highly processed foods that we can gobble down quickly and store readily as fat. At the same time, three-quarters of American diets are lacking in healthy whole foods, such as fruits, vegetables, and dairy, that are slowly digested and help us stay full.

Moreover, most of us are less physically active than our ancestors were—another factor that makes it harder to maintain weight loss. Our bodies were designed to move, and in the process, burn energy. Yet we ride in cars or take the train to work, and we sit at our desks when we get there. Then we spend our weekends watching sports instead of playing them—and too many of us live in neighborhoods that aren't conducive to walking or physical activity. Research has shown that people who have a park, playground, or open space in the neighborhood are 32% less likely to struggle with obesity than those

Lessons from "The Biggest Loser"

To people waging the battle of the bulge, the reality TV show "The Biggest Loser"—recently rebooted after four years off the air—seems to offer tremendous hope. People who struggled with extreme obesity for their entire lives show us on national TV how a grueling diet and hours of intense daily exercise could erase hundreds of pounds of unwanted weight. But 12 years after the show's 2004 debut, we learned that the show's participants may actually be worse off than they were to start with—at least, in some ways.

In a 2016 study published in the journal *Obesity*, researchers followed 14 contestants during and after the show. As expected, their metabolisms slowed over the course of the season, as they shed weight. But that wasn't all. By the final weigh-in, their leptin levels had plummeted, rendering them constantly hungry. Their thyroid function—which governs metabolism and many other bodily functions—had also slowed.

Over the following six years, the combined effects of these hormonal changes conspired to make the contestants regain much, if not all, of the weight they'd lost. But the truly shocking part was that their leptin and metabolism levels never rebounded to what they had been before the show. In fact, the more weight a contestant lost, the slower his or her metabolism became. This explains why weight regain was inevitable, even though they were eating less food than ever.

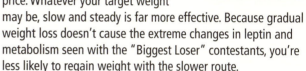

Are there lessons for the rest of us in this experience? Yes and no. In the real world, of course, we're unlikely to shed so many pounds so quickly, since we don't have round-the-clock coaching from doctors, nutritionists, and personal trainers. However, the broader lesson still applies—namely, that drastic weight loss in a short amount of time comes with a price. Whatever your target weight may be, slow and steady is far more effective. Because gradual weight loss doesn't cause the extreme changes in leptin and metabolism seen with the "Biggest Loser" contestants, you're less likely to regain weight with the slower route.

Problems with "The Biggest Loser" approach also suggest that for those who have severe obesity (meaning a body mass index greater than 40; see "Sizing up body weight," page 6), the most effective path to sustained weight loss might not be diet and exercise, even though those are key elements of a healthy lifestyle and important for maintaining weight loss. So far the strongest evidence is for weight-loss surgery (see page 45), which can change the "set point" of weight and metabolism that your body strives to maintain.

who don't have outdoor recreational spaces nearby.

Health experts refer to this combination of too much high-calorie food and too little exercise as an "obesogenic" environment—an environment that encourages us to develop obesity. Plus, there's growing evidence that other aspects of the way we live today—such as how little sleep we get and how much chronic stress we're under—can affect our weight as well, since they affect hormones that govern hunger and satiety.

Why we love to eat

Have you ever wanted a piece of cake or a handful of chips, even though you weren't really hungry? It's not unusual. We're driven to eat by two types of food cues that come through two different systems, one internal and the other external. The internal system, known as your homeostatic system, is guided by your body's need for food to survive. Internal levels of nutrients and hormones, such as leptin and ghrelin, send signals back and forth between the brain and the gut telling you when you're hungry or when you've had enough to eat. This is the system that makes your stomach start growling when you haven't eaten for hours.

The second system, called the hedonic system, is driven by external factors such as liking or wanting food—for instance, when you decide to have a second piece of apple pie on Thanksgiving even though you're already stuffed. Its urges are also responsible for insatiable cravings that make it hard to stop thinking about foods like chocolate, French fries, or pizza.

It's easy to assume that your homeostatic and hedonic hunger systems play equal roles in regulating your food intake. Yet that's hardly the case. Your environment influences the amount of food you eat far more than hunger does. Food that tastes good stimulates your appetite, so you naturally want to keep eating it. In fact, simply liking the way a food tastes can prompt you to eat 44% more of it.

But just because you enjoy the way it tastes, that

doesn't necessarily mean the food satisfies you completely. Research reveals that the longer you eat a food, the less alluring it becomes. That's why you eat more when there is a greater variety of food available. For example, would you rather eat one enormous steak or a steak with a baked potato and a brownie for dessert? If you picked the latter, you've got plenty of company. From an evolutionary perspective, desire for variety ensured that humans would eat a diet with many different foods, providing a healthy range of nutrients. But in today's world, with a seemingly endless supply of foods to choose from, it's easy to overeat simply to satisfy your biological urge for lots of diverse tastes.

Another reason that food doesn't necessarily satisfy is that you may be eating mindlessly while working or checking your Twitter feed. When you're distracted, it's easy to keep reaching into a bag of chips without realizing how much you're consuming—and if you're not paying attention, you're not gaining the full enjoyment you could be getting, so you continue. You might even find that you eat simply because you're bored. Unfortunately, it doesn't take many extra calories each day to lead to weight gain over time.

Is weight gain in your genes?

Our bodies are programmed to store fat and to maintain those fat supplies for times of scarcity. Yet some people seem to put on weight faster than others. The reason could be genetic.

For decades, health experts believed that some people were especially prone to overweight or obesity because they inherited genes that made their bodies particularly efficient at storing fat to ensure survival. Now, researchers recognize that these "thrifty genes" aren't the only ones that may contribute to weight gain. To date, scientists have uncovered 445 different genes that have been linked to some aspect of obesity. For example, certain people are born with a genetic mutation that results in congenital leptin deficiency, which causes severe obesity as early as infancy. People with this condition are a normal weight at birth, but because they don't produce sufficient leptin, they are always hungry and quickly add weight.

Other genes appear to contribute to excess weight by promoting one of the following:
- a slow metabolism and low calorie-burning rate
- a propensity to be physically inactive
- a reduced ability to burn calories from fat
- a tendency to develop excess fat cells and store high levels of body fat.

The power of genetic influences on weight varies substantially from person to person and could account for anywhere from 16% to 40% of the variation in body mass index (BMI), according to studies of twins. In general, if both of your parents or other close blood relatives are significantly overweight, you're much more likely to develop obesity than a person without a family history of overweight. If you have a strong family history of obesity, especially severe obesity, genes are likely involved.

However, biology is not destiny. Even people with the so-called fat mass and obesity-associated (FTO) gene—the first gene discovered that contributes to common types of obesity—are much less likely to be overweight if they engage in a high level of physical activity. Dietary changes can also benefit people with a number of other obesity-related genes. And in some cases, improvements in gut bacteria may even help (see "Gut instinct," page 5). The bottom line is clear: you cannot change your genes, but you can control your environment—and it is the environment we live in that has driven the dramatic increase in obesity since the 1970s.

Food: It's everywhere

We may not notice it, but we're surrounded by food. We nosh on it at movies, sporting events, and the mall; we celebrate with it at the office; and when we're in a hurry, we eat entire meals in the car. Whenever we're the slightest bit hungry, we can buy snacks (and sometimes full meals) from gas stations, convenience stores, drugstores, or vending machines.

But fast food is only part of the equation. Eating out frequently at *any* restaurant can lead to weight gain. In fact, an analysis found that the average entree at non-chain restaurants provided roughly 1,200 calories. That's more than half the calories most women and some men should eat in an entire day. No wonder our average daily intake has jumped by as much as 217 calories (for

> ### Gut instinct
>
> Could the bacteria in your digestive tract affect your body weight? A growing body of research says yes. Your gut is home to more than 100 trillion microbial cells. That's 10 times the number of human cells in your body. These microbes are incredibly diverse, with up to 1,150 different species that can potentially live in your gut. They have all sorts of important jobs, such as regulating immune and digestive health and even influencing your mood. Now, research is finding links between the types of bacteria you harbor and your body weight.
>
> Different microbes have different effects on weight. Some may help you stay slim by stimulating the production of hormones that keep you feeling full, such as leptin. Others may promote weight gain by increasing the fermentation of carbohydrates, encouraging the body to absorb more of their calories. Still other microbes may prompt the body to store greater amounts of fat. In general, the greater the diversity of microbes, the better, since the "good" ones can help counteract the "bad."
>
> The foods you eat and your environment determine your unique gut bacterial profile. A diet containing lots of fiber-filled plant foods appears to protect against obesity-causing bacteria, while the typical Western diet—rife with sugar, fat, and animal products—has been linked to microbes that promote weight gain. Amazingly, it doesn't take long to alter the composition of your gut bacteria. In one Harvard study, researchers found that changes in diet could affect a person's gut microbes in as little as one day.

women) and 491 calories (for men) in the past 40 years.

Even when it's not mealtime, food still seems to beckon. Candy bars and chips are conveniently located right next to the supermarket checkout line. Food advertisements tempt us from magazines, television, social media, and highway billboards. The trouble is, these ads aren't pushing bananas or broccoli. Food marketing often focuses on foods filled with fat, sugar, and sodium, such as fast food and candy. On any given day, children see an average of 15 food commercials on TV. Of these, 98% are for unhealthy foods. Adults aren't immune either, as research finds that watching TV food ads encourages us to eat more, even when we're not particularly hungry. Ironically, if you're on a diet, the sway of these ads is even stronger.

Then there's the increasing availability of cheap food. Price is one of the most powerful factors influencing the amount of food we eat and our obesity risk. Thanks to economies of scale in both farming and distribution, food has become less expensive than ever and, as a result, we're eating more and more of it. Unfortunately, the foods that have become cheapest are often those that we should be eating the least of, namely prepackaged, processed foods that are filled with high-calorie ingredients like fat and sugar. And deep discounts for giant packages of food don't help either, as supersized packaging prompts us to eat 20% to 40% more by distorting our perception of what a reasonable serving size is.

Growing portions aren't just limited to food packages. Since the 1950s, the average restaurant meal has quadrupled in size—and many of us are in the habit of cleaning our plates. In the mid-20th century, a cup of soda was only 7 ounces. Today, you can buy giant cups that are six times as big, clocking in at 42 ounces. Not that long ago, hamburgers were less than 4 ounces. Today, a quarter-pounder looks tiny compared with the 12-ounce burgers served in some restaurants. Even the size of our plates and glasses has ballooned. From 1980 to 2000, the size of the average dinner plate grew from 10 inches to 12 inches. That's a stunning 44% increase in surface area.

Despite mushrooming portion sizes, we rarely notice when there's too much food on our plates. When a serving doubles in size, it only looks about 50% to 70% larger to the human eye. In one study, researchers offered volunteers four different serving sizes of macaroni and cheese. When served the largest portion, the volunteers polished off 30% more food than when given the smallest portion. However, they didn't report feeling any more full than when they ate the smallest size. Even more surprising, 45% of the volunteers didn't realize that they were eating a larger portion. Similarly, drinking from a bigger glass can cause you to increase your intake by 15%.

A nation that's too busy to eat right

The problem isn't just that we're surrounded by tempting snacks that are high in calories and low in nutrition. It's that our entire lifestyles have changed in ways that promote weight gain. We are too stressed, get too little sleep, spend too much time in front of screens, and are often too busy to cook healthy meals.

Time pressures. School, work, and family obligations often lead people to eat on the run. Snacking is not as conducive to good nutrition as preparing healthful meals. Yet today, Americans spend half an hour less cooking each day than they did 50 years ago. For many of us, cooking means popping a frozen meal in the microwave or whipping up pasta from a boxed mix before we race out the door to shuttle our kids to soccer practice, band, or play rehearsal. These ready-made convenience meals tend to be less healthy and lead to more weight gain than meals made from scratch. And when we have an evening in, we're more likely than ever to take advantage of the growing array of food delivery options, so we can enjoy a favorite restaurant meal while we relax in front of the television.

The technology factor. People who spend hours a day looking at screens—whether computers or TVs—are more likely to be obese than those who don't. It's unclear if excessive screen time is a driving factor in obesity; it could be that people with greater body size are more likely to choose sedentary activities. But studies have shown multiple reasons why screen time could lead to weight gain:
- Eating while online or in front of the TV makes you less aware of your body's satiety signals and more likely to keep eating even after you're full.
- When you snack as opposed to eating real sit-down meals, you tend to reach for foods that are less healthful.
- Screen time is sedentary time, so you burn fewer calories.
- TV commercials prompt you to eat when you're not hungry by tempting you with tasty foods.
- Watching TV in the dark makes it difficult to keep track of how much food you're really eating.

Not enough ZZZs. The less you sleep, the more likely you are to be overweight. The link appears to be especially strong among children, according to a review in the journal *Obesity*. Lack of sufficient sleep tends to disrupt hormones that control hunger and appetite. For example, you have higher levels of ghrelin and lower levels of leptin when you are sleep-deprived. You are also more likely to reach for sugary foods to boost your energy—and less motivated to exercise, because you're fatigued.

Stress. Stress is a common thread intertwining some of these factors. For example, the same time pressures that lead to unhealthy eating can also ramp up stress, which has its own effects on weight gain (see "Lower your stress level," page 35). Stress can also cause you to lose sleep. And it can lead to stress eating, in which you crave sugary foods for the measure of comfort they bring, at least temporarily.

Medications that make you gain

Medications you're taking could be causing you to gain weight as well (see Table 1, page 7). For example, certain antipsychotic medications stimulate special histamine receptors in the brain that increase hunger. Often, when people who are using these medications switch to a new drug, their hunger disappears. However, the impact of medication on appetite varies a great deal from person to person, so some people may have no increase in hunger at all. If you suspect your medication is making it difficult for you to lose weight or is causing weight gain, speak with your doctor. He or she may be able to prescribe an alternative drug that is more weight loss–friendly.

Sizing up body weight

It's clear, then, that being overweight isn't a matter of personal failing. But we still need to tackle the consequences. We hear terms like overweight and obesity all the time, but what exactly do these mean? Both of these words are used to describe having more body fat than is optimal for good health; the difference is simply a matter of degree. Either one can lead to chronic diseases like heart disease, diabetes, and gastroesophageal reflux disease and can even shorten your life span.

How do you know which category your weight falls into—normal, overweight, or obesity? Health care professionals use a tool known as body mass index (BMI), an approximate measure of body fat based on a person's height and weight, to determine whether or not that person's weight falls within a healthy range. To find your BMI, you can use a Web-based calcula-

Table 1: Medications that cause weight gain

Ironically, medications you're taking to improve your physical and mental health could be causing you to gain weight.

MEDICATION	USED FOR
Anticonvulsants carbamazepine (Carbatrol, Tegretol) divalproex (Depakote) gabapentin (Neurontin, others) valproic acid (Depakene)	Convulsions and bipolar disorder
Antihistamines azelastine (Astelin, Astepro) cetirizine (Zyrtec) diphenhydramine (Benadryl) fexofenadine (Allegra)	Allergies
Antihypertensives beta blockers: • acebutolol (Sectral) • atenolol (Tenormin) • metoprolol (Lopressor) • propranolol (Inderal) clonidine (Catapres) nisoldipine (Sular)	High blood pressure
Antipsychotics aripiprazole (Abilify, Aristada) clozapine (Clozaril) iloperidone (Fanapt) olanzapine (Zyprexa) paliperidone (Invega) quetiapine (Seroquel) risperidone (Risperdal)	Bipolar disorder and schizophrenia
Chemotherapy anastrozole (Arimidex) tamoxifen (Nolvadex)	Cancer
Corticosteroids cortisone methylprednisone prednisone	Inflammatory diseases such as asthma, rheumatoid arthritis, and lupus
Contraceptives levonorgestrel (Plan B, others) medroxyprogesterone (Provera, Depo-Provera) norethindrone (Ortho Micronor, others)	Birth control
Diabetes drugs chlorpropamide (Diabinese) glipizide (Glucotrol) glyburide (DiaBeta, Glynase, Micronase) insulin pioglitazone (Actos) rosiglitazone (Avandia) tolbutamide (Orinase)	Blood sugar control
Monoamine oxidase inhibitors (MAOIs) phenelzine (Nardil) tranylcypromine (Parnate)	Depression
Mood stabilizer lithium (Eskalith, Lithobid)	Bipolar disorder
Selective serotonin reuptake inhibitors citalopram (Celexa) escitalopram (Lexapro) fluoxetine (Prozac) fluvoxamine (Luvox) paroxetine (Paxil) sertraline (Zoloft)	Depression
Tricyclic antidepressants amitriptyline (Elavil) desipramine (Norpramin, Pertofrane) imipramine (Tofranil) nortriptyline (Pamelor)	Depression

tor, such as the one at www.health.harvard.edu/BMI. A BMI of 25 to 29 is considered overweight. Obesity is defined as a BMI of greater than 30, while severe obesity is a BMI of 40 or higher.

In addition to calculating your BMI, it's helpful to consider where you carry your extra weight. If it settles around your middle—a problem known as abdominal obesity—it can further increase your health risks. That's because fat in the abdomen is more metabolically active than fat stored elsewhere, so it secretes more fatty acids, hormones, and inflammatory compounds into your bloodstream. Health experts define abdominal obesity as a waist circumference measuring 35 inches or more for women or 40 inches or more for men.

The following chapters will show you how to shed those pounds in a healthful way.

The benefits of weight loss

Your body weight has a profound impact on your health. Excess pounds can put you at a higher-than-average risk for at least 195 different health problems (see Figure 1, page 9). These conditions include the nation's leading causes of death—heart disease, stroke, diabetes, high blood pressure, high cholesterol, fatty liver disease, and certain cancers.

On a more immediate level, overweight or obesity makes it a challenge just to get around. The strain of too much weight can make it hard to do tasks that used to be easier, such as walking the dog, carrying groceries, or even getting out of the car. It can also make your joints ache. Every extra pound of weight you carry puts 4 extra pounds of pressure on your knees, making 10 extra pounds feel more like 40.

Losing even a few pounds can make you feel better both mentally and physically, and it can lower your risk of chronic disease. This chapter highlights a few of the most important health benefits.

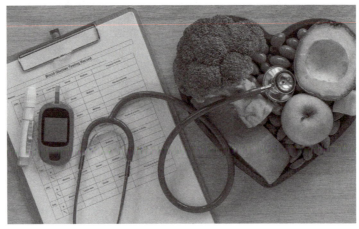

A modest amount of weight loss, achieved through a healthful diet and exercise program, can slash your risk of developing diabetes. If you already have diabetes, it can help you manage the disease.

Diabetes prevention and management

Diabetes occurs when you have too much sugar (glucose) in your bloodstream. Over time, that excess sugar can damage cells and organs, potentially leading to heart disease, kidney failure, blindness, and limb amputation. A staggering 34 million Americans have diabetes, yet more than one in five of them don't even know it—and an additional 88 million have prediabetes, a condition that often leads to diabetes. About 90% of people with type 2 diabetes (the most common form of the disease) are overweight or obese.

The good news is that you can prevent or delay the onset of type 2 diabetes through a combination of weight loss, healthy diet, and exercise. A large trial called the Diabetes Prevention Program found that a modest weight loss of about 7%, achieved through a healthy diet and exercise program, reduced the risk of developing diabetes by 58% in people with prediabetes. That's nearly double the 31% reduction in risk for those taking the diabetes drug metformin (Glucophage).

For people who already have diabetes, weight loss achieved through diet and exercise—together with medication—can help manage diabetes and prevent its devastating complications, including heart attacks.

Less heart disease

Carrying excess weight boosts the risk of developing heart disease. The heavier you are, the greater the risk. The damage is both direct and indirect. On the most obvious level, the strain of all that extra weight means that the heart has to work harder to pump blood throughout the body. Less obviously, overweight increases a number of risk factors for heart disease. For example, it multiplies the risk of high blood pressure (hypertension) approximately threefold, while obesity elevates the risk sixfold.

Weight loss can help reverse the risks. For roughly every pound of weight lost, blood pressure drops an average of 1 point. Shedding 3% to 5% of your body weight—and keeping it off—can reduce fats in the blood known as triglycerides, which are linked to heart disease. And a weight loss of 5% to 10% can improve your cholesterol levels—reducing harmful LDL cholesterol (which contributes to plaque buildup) and boosting helpful HDL (which helps remove plaque from the arteries).

Reduced risk of cancer

When you think of the leading causes of cancer, things like cigarette smoking and family history of the disease probably come to mind. But overweight and obesity also have a tremendous impact on whether you will develop cancer. Types of cancer that have been linked to excess weight include cancers of the breast, colon, esophagus, kidney, liver, pancreas, and uterus.

Figure 1: Medical complications of excess weight

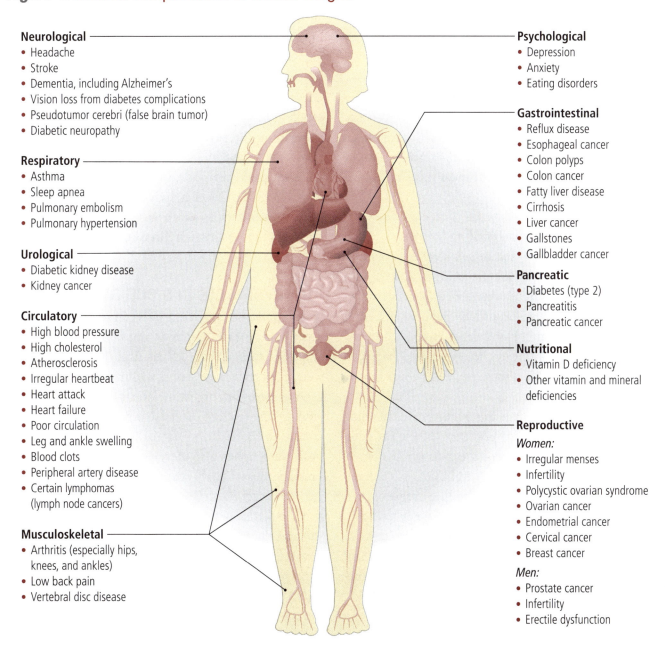

Neurological
- Headache
- Stroke
- Dementia, including Alzheimer's
- Vision loss from diabetes complications
- Pseudotumor cerebri (false brain tumor)
- Diabetic neuropathy

Respiratory
- Asthma
- Sleep apnea
- Pulmonary embolism
- Pulmonary hypertension

Urological
- Diabetic kidney disease
- Kidney cancer

Circulatory
- High blood pressure
- High cholesterol
- Atherosclerosis
- Irregular heartbeat
- Heart attack
- Heart failure
- Poor circulation
- Leg and ankle swelling
- Blood clots
- Peripheral artery disease
- Certain lymphomas (lymph node cancers)

Musculoskeletal
- Arthritis (especially hips, knees, and ankles)
- Low back pain
- Vertebral disc disease

Psychological
- Depression
- Anxiety
- Eating disorders

Gastrointestinal
- Reflux disease
- Esophageal cancer
- Colon polyps
- Colon cancer
- Fatty liver disease
- Cirrhosis
- Liver cancer
- Gallstones
- Gallbladder cancer

Pancreatic
- Diabetes (type 2)
- Pancreatitis
- Pancreatic cancer

Nutritional
- Vitamin D deficiency
- Other vitamin and mineral deficiencies

Reproductive

Women:
- Irregular menses
- Infertility
- Polycystic ovarian syndrome
- Ovarian cancer
- Endometrial cancer
- Cervical cancer
- Breast cancer

Men:
- Prostate cancer
- Infertility
- Erectile dysfunction

Excess weight increases a person's risk of at least 195 different medical conditions that affect all the major systems of the body. One of the most common is type 2 diabetes, which can lead to serious complications in the heart, kidneys, nerves, and eyes.

There are a number of possible explanations for the cancer connection. Fat cells—especially those that accumulate around your waist (abdominal fat)—are metabolically active, producing a variety of substances that increase low-grade chronic inflammation. This inflammation can promote tumor development. It can also damage DNA, causing mutations that allow cancer cells to multiply unchecked. And it can stimulate angiogenesis—the growth of new blood vessels that feed tumors with oxygen and nutrients. All these processes help fuel cancer growth. The larger the fat cells—and the more you have—the more of these inflammatory substances you have circulating in your body. Studies suggest that as many as 20% of cancers begin as a direct result of inflammation.

What's more, a sedentary lifestyle, which frequently goes hand in hand with a higher BMI, can also raise your odds of cancer. According to the American Institute for Cancer Research, simply walking more and sitting less can lower your cancer risk.

Protection for the liver

Most people are aware that excess alcohol consumption can harm the liver, but the leading cause of liver damage in this country is non-alcoholic fatty liver disease (NAFLD). NAFLD usually happens in people who have obesity, high blood sugar, high blood pressure, or abnormal levels of cholesterol and triglycerides in their blood. All of these problems contribute to excess fat in the liver.

From there, things can spiral downward. In about one in 20 people with NAFLD, fat in the liver triggers chronic liver inflammation—a condition known as non-alcoholic steatohepatitis, or NASH. This inflammation can scar the liver tissue, leading in severe cases to cirrhosis. The result can be liver failure or liver cancer, either of which may require a liver transplant.

The best treatment for NASH is weight loss. One major study showed that a 10% weight loss can reduce liver fat and inflammation and possibly reduce existing scarring.

Less reflux

Everybody has heartburn from time to time, but when it is an issue two or more times a week, it's known as gastroesophageal reflux disease (GERD). A surprising 20% of Americans have this condition. GERD happens when the sphincter that seals off your stomach from your esophagus weakens and opens, allowing corrosive stomach acid to flow backward into your esophagus. Because overweight or obesity puts extra pressure on your middle, it can make you more likely to develop GERD. Untreated, chronic GERD can lead to a syndrome known as Barrett's esophagus, which is marked by changes in the esophageal lining. In severe cases, Barrett's esophagus can progress to cancer.

The good news is that losing weight can help control GERD. Other helpful changes include eating smaller meals, avoiding alcohol and caffeine, and eating dinner at least two to three hours before bedtime.

Improvements in sleep apnea

Sleep apnea—a condition in which a person temporarily stops breathing many times during the night—affects at least 2% to 3% of Americans. Too much weight, particularly around your middle and neck, can interfere with nighttime breathing, making people who are overweight or obese especially prone to this condition. In addition to leading to daytime sleepiness, sleep apnea also elevates the risk of high blood pressure, heart attack, stroke, and diabetes.

However, weight loss can help. A study published in *Sleep Medicine* found that volunteers with both obesity and sleep apnea who lost 8½ pounds experienced fewer apnea episodes and reduced the progression of the disease by 80%.

The essential ingredients of a healthy diet

Few things are more confusing than weight-loss advice. Online or in your favorite magazines, you'll find loads of articles on both diet and exercise. But which is really better for weight loss? While both are important for *maintaining* weight loss, experts agree that diet is far more powerful than exercise when it comes to losing weight in the first place. Of course, exercise does play a role (see "Why moving matters" on page 32)—and it has myriad health benefits—but it takes more work than you might think to burn off a lot of calories. It's much easier to trim 150 calories by, say, skipping a 12-ounce soda. That's why developing a healthy eating strategy should be your first line of defense. This chapter will help you get started.

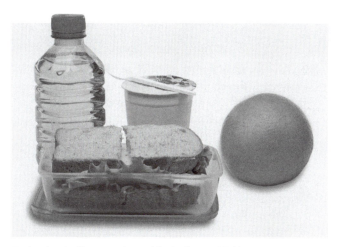

Pack a lunch, if you work outside the home. Making your own lunches will allow you to control portion sizes and limit tasty (but caloric) add-ons like, mayo, butter, and sugar.

How fast should you overhaul your diet?

It's easy to assume the fastest way to reach your desired weight is by giving your diet a complete and drastic overhaul. However, many people find that it's easier to make a series of small changes one by one, giving themselves plenty of time and flexibility to reach their goals. The benefit of this strategy is that it allows you to eat many of the same foods you love and gradually master changes in your eating habits that will hopefully last for years to come.

If that sounds appealing, try setting a six-month goal of reducing your body weight by 5% to 10%. Start by making a list of mini-goals that you think you can realistically achieve over time. Once you've mastered one, maintain it while you try another, and another. Before you know it, you'll be eating more healthfully and the pounds will slowly start to fall off. If you're not sure where to begin, these suggestions can help:

Cook dinner at least three times a week. When you cook, you control the portion size and the ingredients. To get started, try some of the quick and healthy recipes in the Special Section starting on page 21.

Brown-bag it at least three times a week. You'll save hundreds of calories and money, too. To make it easy, pack up home-cooked leftovers right after dinner for lunch the next day.

Add two healthy foods to your shopping list every week. On the pages that follow, you'll learn about all kinds of foods that can keep you full and reduce hunger. Aim to try a minimum of two of these each week. If you don't know what to do with these foods once you buy them, search for recipes online.

Rethink your drink. Eliminating soda and replacing it with water has been shown to help people shed 2.5% of their body weight in just six months. Other options include coffee without sugar, unsweetened iced tea, or sparkling water. For a pop of flavor in your water, add cucumber slices, whole fresh berries, or a wedge of grapefruit, orange, lemon, or lime. (If you're wondering about artificial sweeteners, see "What about diet soft drinks?" on page 12.)

Try a new spin on fast food. If you regularly eat fast food, you don't have to avoid it entirely. Instead, scout out the restaurant's website for some of the lighter options on the menu. Fast-food outlets and other quick-service restaurants are responding to con-

What about diet soft drinks?

Can artificially sweetened beverages help you lose weight? The research is mixed. Some studies show that these drinks can help with long-term weight loss. Others hint that they may cause weight gain. Still others indicate that they make little difference either way.

One reason these beverages may not help much is that people often use them to try to offset other high-calorie foods—for example, drinking a diet soda to wash down a cheeseburger and fries. But other mechanisms may be at play, too. A growing body of evidence suggests that artificial sweeteners wreak havoc on the balance of healthy bacteria in the gut, favoring the growth of certain types of bacteria that lead you to absorb more calories from the food you eat (see "Gut instinct," page 5). In addition, some health experts are concerned about their impact on appetite. When you eat sweet foods, your brain naturally expects calories to follow. Because artificially sweetened foods and drinks supply sweetness without the calories of sugar, they may confuse your brain into thinking you need to keep eating to get those missing calories, rather than satisfying hunger the way a small amount of sugar would.

The bottom line: If you're eating a diet of healthful, natural foods, there's no need to feel guilty about the occasional diet soda, but try to avoid it as a daily habit.

---

sumer preferences by offering more healthy options.

Avoid ultra-high-calorie foods. Some foods supply so many calories that they make weight loss nearly impossible. See Table 6 on page 20 for examples of foods to avoid when eating out.

Once you've got the hang of it, you can increase your targets—cook dinner five times a week, for example, and remake your shopping list, replacing unhealthy foods with healthier ones.

Moving beyond calorie counting

For decades, experts believed counting calories was the key to dropping unwanted pounds, and calorie lists regularly appeared in books and magazines and online. Now, experts realize strict calorie counting isn't the best strategy. "Over the long term, your weight is controlled more by biology than willpower," says Dr. David Ludwig, professor of nutrition at the Harvard T.H. Chan School of Public Health. "You can cut back calories and lose weight temporarily, but your body pushes back with rising hunger and slowing metabolism."

Experts are also now learning that not all calories are created equal when it comes to weight loss. Some foods can keep you far more satisfied than others, helping you eat less over all. You'll learn more about those foods later in this report—in particular, about finding foods with a low caloric density, which is not the same thing as just counting up the total number of calories. Finally, when you rely solely on counting calories, you never learn to listen to your body's inner hunger and satiety signals, which can be powerful tools in helping to keep unwanted pounds off for good (see "Slow down—and try mindful eating," page 31).

That's not to say calories don't matter at all. Experts still agree that consuming fewer calories than you burn leads to weight loss. But you don't need to obsess about them. Instead, it can be more helpful to have a general idea of how many calories you should limit yourself to in a day—and which foods are more likely to help you stay within that range. Think of it as *calorie awareness*, as opposed to calorie counting.

For example, a matcha green tea smoothie might sound like a healthy choice. But if you were to order a large matcha smoothie at a typical juice bar, you'd be drinking 540 calories in one sitting—more than a third of your entire daily energy allotment, assuming you're on a 1,500-calorie-a-day diet. If you were to choose a small smoothie instead, you would cut that number almost in half, to 300 calories. Simply being aware of the calories in the smoothie might make you opt for the smaller size. That's how calorie awareness can help.

In this report, you'll occasionally see calorie counts listed for foods. Don't feel that you need to use this information to tally up every bite you take. Instead, consider it a reference to help you gain a general understanding of the impact of certain foods—and their serving sizes—on your weight-loss efforts.

How many calories do you burn in a day?

A calorie is a measure of the energy that your body

can derive from certain foods and nutrients. On the most basic level, your body uses this energy for three things:

1. To maintain your basal metabolism (50% to 65% of calories). Your basal metabolic rate, or BMR, is the rate at which your body burns energy for basic functions, such as breathing or making your heart beat, as well as building cells, hormones, and antibodies. Because BMR depends on factors such as age, sex, body weight, muscle mass, and genetic makeup, it can vary substantially from person to person.

2. To fuel physical activity (30% to 50% of calories). Whether you're walking the dog or running a marathon, your body requires energy to move. The longer and more strenuous your activity, the greater your calorie burn. Even small movements such as fidgeting can increase your energy expenditure (see "That's NEAT!" on page 33).

3. To digest food and absorb nutrients (10% of calories). This calorie-requiring process is known as the thermic effect of food.

There are many complicated equations for estimating your calorie needs, but they're really not necessary. Online calculators, such as the Body Weight Planner from the National Institute of Diabetes and Digestive and Kidney Diseases—which you can access at www.niddk.nih.gov/bwp—can give you a good estimate. For optimal weight loss, many experts recommend a range of 1,200 to 1,500 calories a day for the average woman who does not have severe obesity and 1,500 to 1,800 calories a day for the average man. While you may be tempted to eat less than this for faster weight loss, it's very difficult to meet your nutrient needs with fewer than 1,200 daily calories per day.

Beating hunger with a high-quality diet

Anyone who's tried dieting knows that one big obstacle is hunger. But you don't have to starve yourself to reach your target. It's easy to assume that large servings are necessary to keep you full and that small ones will leave you hungry. Yet there are many other factors that go into a food's satisfaction quotient. For example, have you ever eaten an entire bag of pretzels, only to find that your stomach started to rumble a couple of hours later? Despite the ample serving size, the pretzels themselves weren't all that filling. On the flip side, think about eating nuts. Unlike pretzels, nuts are highly satiating, so it's unlikely you'd ever be inclined to polish off an entire bag.

The difference between these two foods boils down to *quality*, which reflects the ingredients and nutrients that make up a food. Pretzels are made from processed carbohydrates, starches that have essentially been broken down by a machine so your body doesn't have to work hard to digest them. These types of carbs are also found in foods such as white bread, mashed potatoes, pancakes, sugar-sweetened cereals, and—of course—desserts. After you eat them, they flood your bloodstream with sugar, giving you a quick shot of energy that temporarily quells hunger.

Your body learns to seek out these treats whenever hunger kicks in. The trouble is, this can turn into a vicious circle, in which these rapidly digested carbs make you feel better for a short while, but soon you end up hungry all over again and begin to crave them even more. How does that happen? "Eating processed carbohydrates raises insulin levels, and insulin drives calories into fat cells for storage," says Dr. Ludwig. "So a few hours later, fat cells

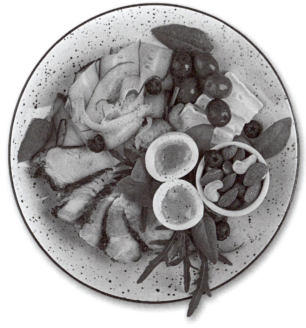

You don't have to starve yourself to reach your target weight. Meals that include lean protein, healthy fats, and fiber-rich unprocessed carbohydrates can help you feel full.

Sleuthing out added sugars

There's one carbohydrate that just about everyone could use less of, and that's sugar. The average American eats an incredible 20 teaspoons of sugar every day. In addition to making blood glucose and insulin soar, sugar loads you down with empty calories that take the place of important nutrients you need to look and feel your best.

Still, not all sugars are the same. Sugar comes in two forms—natural sugars, such as the type found in fruit, and the added sugars that you'll find in many processed foods. Naturally occurring sugars aren't much of a concern, as these usually come packaged in small doses along with important nutrients such as vitamins, minerals, antioxidants, and fiber. Added sugars, on the other hand, have no nutritional benefit, and a growing body of research suggests they encourage obesity and diabetes.

Identifying products with added sugars has become much easier thanks to recent changes to the Nutrition Facts panel on most food labels. The new panel separates out added sugars from total sugars. If the amount of added sugar surprises you, remember that sugar can masquerade under less obvious names, like corn syrup, molasses, sucrose, and dextrose.

Even seemingly healthy foods can have worrisome amounts of sugar. Table 2, below, lists some of the biggest offenders.

Table 2: Sneaky sources of sugar

FOOD	SUGAR (teaspoons*)
Blueberry muffin, 1 medium	9
Dried cranberries, sweetened, ¼ cup	7¼
Coleslaw, 1 cup	5¾
Baked beans, 1 cup	5
Greek yogurt, strawberry flavor, 5.3 ounces	4
Granola, ½ cup	3
Instant oatmeal, maple brown sugar flavor, 1 packet	3
Barbeque sauce, 2 tablespoons	2¾
Spaghetti sauce, ½ cup	1½

*4 grams of sugar equals 1 teaspoon of sugar.
Source: USDA FoodData Central.

have feasted, but there aren't enough calories in the bloodstream to fuel metabolism." Unfortunately, your brain doesn't always know that there are too many calories trapped in your fat cells. It just senses that there aren't enough in your bloodstream, so it tells you to eat, even though you have plenty of energy on tap.

To make matters worse, highly processed foods don't take much work to chew, making it easy to eat a lot of them in a hurry. Minimally processed whole foods such as nuts, on the other hand, are more dense and solid, so chewing them takes a lot of work. Plus, they're filled with nutrients, such as protein, fiber, and healthy fats, that your digestive system must dismantle piece by piece. That process takes time, so these foods hang around longer, helping to ward off hunger.

A 2019 study found that people ate about 500 more calories per day on a diet of ultra-processed foods than they did when they were eating unprocessed foods. Unfortunately, seemingly healthy foods often have surprising amounts of added sugar. For tips on spotting those foods, see "Sleuthing out added sugars" at left.

Good carbohydrates

Although processed carbohydrates can lead to weight gain, not all carbohydrates are bad. In fact, carbohydrate-heavy foods such as peas, beans, lentils, fruits, vegetables, and whole grains can be a healthy part of your weight-loss plan. That's because these whole foods are rich in fiber, a type of calorie-free carbohydrate that your body can't digest. You may have already heard that fiber is beneficial for digestive health. But it's also key for weight management, because it slows down digestion, so a food's other carbohydrates enter your bloodstream more gradually and provide prolonged energy. What's more, in your gut, fiber swells like a sponge, filling you up without adding calories. It's so powerful that one study found that people who ate about 25 grams of fiber a day, without making any other changes to their diets, shed 4.5 pounds in a year.

One of the easiest ways to sneak more fiber into your diet is to increase your intake of whole grains. People who regularly eat whole grains tend to have lower BMIs and less body fat than those who don't eat whole grains. Aim for at least three servings every day.

For more ideas on boosting fiber, see "10 easy tricks to sneak more fiber into your meals" at right.

Fruits and vegetables help with weight loss for a second reason, too: they are low in energy density. Energy density is basically the number of calories in a given weight of food. Because fruits and vegetables typically contain a lot of water, they are big on volume, so they fill you up, yet they're low in calories. They also happen to be some of the healthiest foods out there, so they naturally boost the quality of your diet.

To appreciate the impact of foods with a low energy density, imagine you were deciding between strawberries and potato chips for a snack. Strawberries contain only 10 calories per ounce. An ounce of potato chips delivers 150 calories. So for the same number of calories, you could eat either 1 ounce of potato chips (about 22 chips) or 15 ounces of strawberries (roughly three cups). By choosing the food with the lower energy density—the strawberries—you would be able to eat more food for fewer calories and feel fuller. For easy tips to help you downsize the energy density of your meals, see "Tips to help lighten your meals" on page 19.

Lean protein

Protein has been getting a lot of positive attention for its role in weight management, and with good reason. Protein is more satiating than either carbohydrates or fat, so eating a little more protein in place of either of these nutrients can help you feel full longer. How so? On the most basic level, protein is digested gradually, so it sticks with you for hours. But there's more. When you eat protein-rich foods, such as chicken or fish, your gut releases a flood of satiety hormones such as glucagon-like peptide 1 (GLP-1) and peptide YY (PYY), which send out signals to your brain that help control appetite. Protein also offers another bonus. This nutrient takes more energy to digest than carbohydrates or fat, so your body is less likely to squirrel away as many of its calories as fat. That's why weight-loss experts recommend including one serving of protein at every meal (for suggestions, see Table 3, page 16).

Just keep in mind that when it comes to protein, not all forms are on equal footing. Protein from red meat like hamburgers, steaks, and pork or lamb

> ### 10 easy tricks to sneak more fiber into your meals
>
> It's not hard to boost your fiber intake. It's just a matter of becoming aware of sources. (Hint: They're not only in whole grains.)
>
> 1. Add half a cup of blueberries (4 grams fiber) to whole-grain cereal.
> 2. Tuck half a cup of pinto beans (7.5 grams fiber) into a burrito.
> 3. Substitute a cup of quinoa (5 grams fiber) for white rice.
> 4. Toss half a cup of cooked barley (3 grams fiber) into a salad.
> 5. Blend a tablespoon of chia seeds (4 grams fiber) into a smoothie.
> 6. Swap in a cup of whole-wheat spaghetti (5 grams fiber) for regular spaghetti.
> 7. Stir a tablespoon of flaxseed (2 grams fiber) into oatmeal.
> 8. Swap in a cup of bran flakes (7 grams fiber) for cornflakes.
> 9. Substitute a whole-wheat English muffin (4 grams fiber) for a regular English muffin.
> 10. Add half a cup of peas (4 grams fiber) to pasta.

chops usually comes packaged with a hefty dose of saturated fat, a type of fat that is linked to heart disease. Some research even suggests that this type of fat may increase the risk of diabetes. And processed luncheon meats such as deli chicken, ham, or turkey may be even more problematic. Research suggests that the nitrates and nitrites that are added to these foods to preserve freshness and color may lead to insulin resistance. What's more, in late 2015, an international panel of experts convened by the World Health Organization concluded that processed meat raises the risk of colon cancer. Instead, stick with healthier options such as chicken, fish, eggs, tofu, beans, and lentils, which contain less saturated fat.

Healthy fats

For decades, fat was considered to be weight-loss Enemy No. 1. Now, we're learning that a little fat can be helpful, as long as it's the right kind. Like protein, fat is digested slowly, so it keeps you sated. Plus, it makes food taste better, so it can help keep you from feeling deprived. But just as with other nutrients, there are both healthy and unhealthy types of fat. Even though saturated fats spell trouble, other types

Table 3: Healthiest protein sources

From tuna to tofu, protein is found in lots of foods. Here are the healthiest ways to get your fill.

FOOD	PROTEIN (grams)	FAT (grams)	SATURATED FAT (grams)	CALORIES
Chicken breast (grilled, skinless), 3 ounces	26	3	1	128
Salmon steak (cooked), 3 ounces	22	7	1	155
Greek yogurt (nonfat), 6 ounces	17	0	0	100
Tuna fish (canned in water), 3 ounces	17	1	0	73
Tofu (firm), ½ cup	11	5	1	98
Beans, ½ cup	8	0	0	114
Milk (nonfat), 1 cup	8	0	0	83
Peanut butter, 2 tablespoons	7	16	3	191
Almonds, 1 ounce	6	14	1	164
Egg (large), 1	6	5	2	72

Source: USDA FoodData Central.

of fats—called monounsaturated and polyunsaturated fats—are heart-friendly. You can find these beneficial nutrients in olive, canola, sunflower, and safflower oils as well as in avocados, nuts, seeds, olives, and fatty fish such as salmon and sardines.

How much fat is enough, and how much is too much? Health experts now agree that anywhere from 20% to 35% of calories from fat is fine as long as the bulk of these are helpful mono- and polyunsaturated fats. Just bear in mind that a little bit goes a long way, as a given amount of fat contains more than twice the calories of the same amount of carbohydrates or protein.

Low-calorie liquids

Eating more filling, high-quality foods can be a smart strategy. Yet it's easy to overlook a hidden culprit in weight gain: beverages. Fluids account for a hefty 20% of the average American's total calories. That might not sound like cause for alarm, but liquid calories don't send the same feelings of satiety to your brain as solid ones do. That's why nibbling on a small wedge of cheese can help you feel satisfied for a few hours, but drinking a glass of milk doesn't do the trick for very long.

And it's not just a question of total calories—it's also the quality of those calories. More than a third of the average American's liquid calories come from sugary drinks such as soda, fruit drinks, and energy drinks—and presweetened beverages contain far more sugar than you'd ever add yourself. For example, a teaspoon of sugar in your iced tea at home doesn't come close to the 9½ teaspoons (and 150 calories) that you'd get from a 12-ounce can of presweetened tea. The result of all this liquid sugar? People who regularly drink sugary beverages are 55% more likely to be overweight or obese than those who rarely choose these beverages. And those who sip even one or two cans of soda a day are 26% more likely to develop diabetes than infrequent soda drinkers.

Diet drinks may help you transition away from sugar-sweetened beverages, but they won't necessarily help you lose weight, and may come with problems of their own (see "What about diet soft drinks?" on page 12).

What should you do instead? The answer is as close as your kitchen tap. Plain or sparkling water is a much better choice. If that seems too boring, try jazzing it up with slices of lemon, lime, orange, or grapefruit. A sprig of fresh mint or a few raspberries can also add a pleasing hint of flavor. Or brew coffee or tea—just remember to go easy on the cream and sugar.

In addition to slashing calories, drinking two cups of water before a meal could help you eat less. In one study, researchers asked 14 men to eat a breakfast of oatmeal until they were full. One week later, the researchers repeated the experiment, but this time asked the volunteers to drink a pint of water before eating the identical meal. The results? When the men drank the water, they consumed 22% fewer calories. One reason water may tame appetite is that it stretches your stomach, sending signals of fullness to your brain.

Rethinking your plate

Knowing the best sources of carbohydrates, fat, and protein is a good start. But for most people, the difficulty comes in translating that knowledge into actual meals. Habits die hard, and few are as ingrained as dietary choices. When you get to the grocery store, it's tempting to load up your basket the way you normally do. And even buying healthy, weight loss–friendly food is no guarantee that it won't languish for weeks in your refrigerator when you get it home. Just because you know that tilapia is healthier than fried chicken doesn't mean that you know how to prepare it in a tasty way.

The suggestions in this chapter will help you start rethinking what you put on your plate—and will offer easy ways to assemble common ingredients into low-calorie meals without a lot of work.

Make every meal a success

Each meal is an opportunity to eat better. But sometimes it's tricky to know what to choose, especially if you're eating on the run or have little time to cook. That's where it helps to have a strategy. This meal-by-meal guide will help you make the best choices all day long.

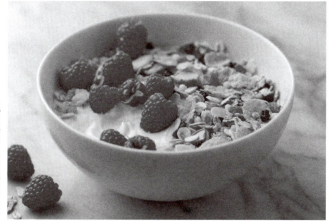

A breakfast of whole-grain cereal with milk, nuts, and berries provides a healthful, well-rounded meal to start your day. The mix of protein, healthy fats, and fiber can help keep you feeling full.

Power up your morning

Breakfast can help you start your day on the right track. Yet many Americans skip this important meal—and that could be hindering their weight-loss efforts. Here's why: breakfast can supply lots of foods and nutrients that are linked to less hunger. Plus, eating more of your calories earlier in the day may help control your appetite later on, so you eat less over all.

But breakfast doesn't have to be a large meal. Work some extra fiber into your day by grabbing a whole-grain English muffin and a single-serving container of yogurt as you run out the door. Or, if you have a few extra minutes, pour yourself a bowl of whole-grain cereal. The milk you add can help prevent midmorning hunger pangs. Or have an egg. With its protein and fat, an egg breakfast is so filling that it's been shown to help people eat less hours later, at lunch and even at dinner.

You might also try one of these quick morning meals, all of which contain protein, fiber, and healthy fat and carbs:

- 1 cup bran flakes with 1 cup sliced strawberries, 1 cup nonfat milk, and 1 tablespoon chopped walnuts (320 calories)
- 1 slice whole-wheat toast with 1 tablespoon peanut butter and 1 sliced apple (290 calories)
- 1 cup cooked old-fashioned or steel-cut oatmeal, 6 ounces plain nonfat Greek yogurt, and ½ cup fresh (or thawed frozen) raspberries (280 calories)
- 1 scrambled egg, ½ cup cantaloupe cubes, and 1 whole-wheat English muffin with 1 tablespoon whipped cream cheese (320 calories)

quicktip | Dish out food in the kitchen rather than placing serving dishes on the dining room table. Keeping serving dishes off the table has been shown to decrease the amount of food people eat by 20% to 29%.

- 1 cup 1% cottage cheese, 1 banana, and 1 tablespoon sliced almonds (300 calories).

Plan for a healthier lunch

If you're like many people, you probably don't even think about lunch until you're beyond hungry. The trouble is, by then, you're desperate to grab whatever you can get your hands on, so you may not always end up making the best choices. In a perfect world, you'd prepare lunch yourself, so you'd always have a nutritious meal right at your fingertips. Of course, if you work outside the home, that's not always possible. Luckily, you can still eat a healthy midday meal, even if you don't have time to brown-bag it.

Rather than waiting until you're famished, it helps to know what to order ahead of time. Get started by gathering a few menus from your favorite take-out restaurants. Then, take a few minutes to highlight the lowest-calorie choices. (If you can check out the nutrition information on the restaurant's website, even better.) Next, stash the menus in a nearby desk drawer. Every morning, when you arrive at your desk, take a minute to set a reminder on your computer or smartphone to go off about 15 minutes before you'd like to have lunch. That way you'll have time to order before you become overly hungry.

Next time you order in—or go out for—lunch, try one of these. They're low in calories and also contain lean protein to keep you full all afternoon long:

- vegetarian burrito bowl made with brown rice, black or pinto beans, onions, peppers, tomato salsa, and shredded lettuce (380 calories)
- turkey sandwich on a 6-inch whole-wheat sub roll with lettuce, tomato, onion, cucumber, olive oil, and vinegar (380 calories)
- Chinese ginger chicken with broccoli (no rice) (300 calories)
- six-piece California roll and six-piece spicy tuna roll (440 calories)
- a bowl of turkey chili (260 calories).

You might be wondering if it wouldn't just be easier to grab a protein bar or prepackaged shake. After all, they don't spoil, plus you can eat them any time it's convenient. Research reveals that meal replacements can be effective weight-loss tools, although

> **quicktip** | Eat only in the kitchen or dining room. A study of 338 parents and children found that those who did this tended to weigh less than members of families who ate in other parts of the house.

some people do not find them sufficiently satisfying, and some brands add too much refined sugar. If you do choose to go the bar or shake route, be sure to read the label carefully, as these products can vary substantially in the quality of their ingredients. Look for bars or shakes that contain

- 300 to 400 calories
- at least 5 grams of fiber
- at least 15 grams of protein
- less than 35% of calories from fat and no more than 10% of calories from saturated fat
- no more than 15 grams of sugar.

Make dinner in a snap

Given the choice, who wouldn't prefer a home-cooked meal to a frozen dinner or take-out? Getting dinner on the table doesn't have to take hours—as long as you have the right game plan. You've already learned the upside of stocking your kitchen with the right ingredients. But making healthy dinners happen starts before that. The key is planning out a few meals that you can prepare—and clean up—quickly. In addition to the

Table 4: Liquid calories

Calories from fluids can add up quickly. These stats can help you keep liquid calories under control.

DRINK	AMOUNT	CALORIES
Sports drink	16-ounce bottle	100
Apple juice	8 ounces	114
Sweetened lemon iced tea	12-ounce bottle	120
Beer	12-ounce bottle	140
White wine	6 ounces	144
Cola	12-ounce can	150
Red wine	6 ounces	155
Gin and tonic	8 ounces	191
Latte (made with whole milk)	16 ounces	220

dinner suggestions in our meal plan (see the Special Section, beginning on page 21), consider these easy meals, which should take no more than 15 minutes to prepare:

- 3 ounces grilled salmon over 3 cups baby spinach tossed with 2 tablespoons Asian sesame vinaigrette salad dressing (350 calories)
- 1 microwave-baked sweet potato topped with 1 cup canned black beans, ½ cup plain nonfat Greek yogurt, and ¼ cup salsa (390 calories)
- 1 two-egg mushroom, onion, and tomato omelet with 1 cup fresh fruit salad (360 calories)
- 1 turkey burger on 1 whole-wheat bun with 1 cup cherry tomatoes tossed with 1 tablespoon balsamic vinaigrette dressing (410 calories)
- 1 cup cooked whole-wheat pasta with ½ cup tomato sauce, ½ cup chopped spinach, ½ cup cannellini beans, and 1 tablespoon Parmesan cheese (370 calories).

Table 5: The best choices when you eat out

Almost every restaurant has some healthy choices on the menu. When in doubt, try these lower-calorie picks.

TYPE OF RESTAURANT	FOOD	APPROXIMATE CALORIES PER SERVING
American	Garden salad with grilled chicken (lunch portion)	400
Chinese	Stir-fried tofu and vegetables, with brown rice	450
Japanese	Hibachi chicken meal (without rice or sauces)	385
Mexican	Chicken tacos on corn tortillas with green peppers, onions, and tomato salsa	425
Pizza	Veggie pizza slice	230

Sources: Company websites for TGI Friday's, P.F. Chang's, Benihana, Chipotle, Pizza Hut.

Tips to help lighten your meals

Even though homemade is best, the foods you cook in your kitchen sometimes contain hidden calories, too. These tricks can help you slim down your meals without sacrificing an ounce of flavor:

- Dial down the meat and bump up the vegetables in soups, stews, casseroles, and pasta sauces.
- Cut the amount of butter or oil you'd usually use in half. Try this with cheese, too.
- Swap in vegetables such as broccoli, tomatoes, or mushrooms for half your pasta or lasagna noodles.
- Try penne or ziti instead of spaghetti. Because these pasta shapes are tubular, they're less dense and contain more air; therefore, they have fewer calories per cup.
- Swap in panko (Japanese-style breadcrumbs) for regular breadcrumbs. It's about 220 calories per cup, versus about twice that for a cup of some brands of breadcrumbs.
- Buy reduced-fat shredded cheese instead of full-fat versions.
- Substitute black beans for half the meat in tacos, chili, or sloppy joes.
- Add finely chopped mushrooms to meatloaf or burgers.
- Make your own salad dressing with two parts vinegar to one part canola or olive oil.

Parents should try to model balanced, healthy eating for their children. Encourage the kids to taste new foods. And don't make them clean their plates if they're not hungry.

A special note for parents

Actions you take—or don't take—today can help your kids have a healthier relationship with food (and a healthier weight) years, or even decades, from now. For example, if you encourage your kids to clean their plates, stop. All this does is teach kids to eat when they aren't hungry, and to not trust their natural hunger and fullness signals. It can be helpful to adopt a "division of responsibility" philosophy—parents decide when meals will happen and what foods will be served, kids

Table 6: Restaurant foods to avoid

Restaurant meals almost always deliver more calories than home-cooked ones. Calories per dish can also vary substantially from restaurant to restaurant depending on serving size and how the food is prepared.

FOOD	APPROXIMATE CALORIES PER SERVING
Fried Chinese dishes such as orange chicken, General Tso's chicken, sesame chicken, and sweet-and-sour chicken or pork	1,578–1,765
Taco salad	906
Lo mein	897
Lasagna	845
Cheese quesadilla	754
Mozzarella sticks	796
Chicken parmesan	614
Onion rings	600

Source: USDA FoodData Central.

It also helps to know that just about anything you order is going to be at least two to three times larger than it should be. Here's how you can avoid overindulging:

- Be on the lookout for menu buzzwords such as "crispy," "battered," or "smothered," which hint that a dish is deep-fried or drowning in sauce.
- Split an entree with a friend. Or order an appetizer and soup or salad instead of a full meal.
- At the start of your meal, ask your server to place half your meal in a to-go box.
- Steer clear of buffet-style or all-you-can-eat restaurants. Their endless choices and unlimited quantities practically beg you to overeat.

Don't be shy about asking lots of questions about how your food is prepared. It's also okay to make special requests for lighter preparation—such as asking for fish broiled or grilled instead of deep-fried or sautéed—or for dressings and sauces to be served on the side, so you can control how much you add to your meal.

decide which and how much of the foods offered they want to eat. Kids may be hungrier some days—like when they are going through a growth spurt—and less hungry other days. Try to model balanced, varied eating for your kids, encourage them to taste new foods, and encourage them to eat the kinds of foods that give them energy to play and be active. For more on raising healthy eaters, you can visit the website of the nonprofit Ellyn Satter Institute (www.ellynsatterinstitute.org).

Smarter strategies for dining out

Realistically, everyone has to eat out sometimes. The good news is that restaurants are increasingly offering healthier options (see Table 5, page 19). You just need to know what to look for, as well as what to avoid, especially since restaurant offerings frequently include much more butter, cream, and oil—and therefore calories—than foods prepared at home (see Table 6, above). Even seemingly diet-friendly options, such as salad bars, can present hazards if you ladle on the ranch dressing, scoop up the croutons and bacon bits, and fill your plate with "pasta salad." (Pasta is not salad, even if it contains a few diced vegetables.)

The art of snacking

You may have heard that eating lots of small meals or snacks is the best way to curb your appetite. The truth is, this advice has been greatly exaggerated. While it's true that eating only once or twice a day can make you hungrier, nibbling all day long won't reduce hunger or help you eat less.

If you have to go for a long stretch between meals, a balanced snack is fine. The trick is to choose one that contains some protein, fiber, or a little bit of healthy fat for lasting staying power. At the same time, you'll want to avoid those that are made of overly processed carbohydrates that do little to sustain you, such as chips, cookies, sugary drinks, and crackers made from white flour—these rapidly absorbed carbohydrates do little to keep you full compared with whole foods that are slowly digested.

When choosing snacks, simply follow the same guidelines as you do for meals—prioritize whole foods with minimal processing, and look for the healthiest sources of fat, carbs, and protein. For ideas, see "Snacks" on page 23.

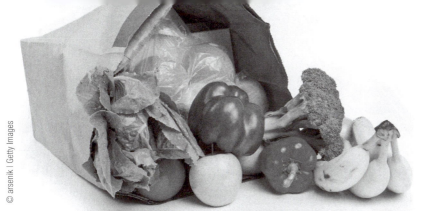

SPECIAL SECTION

What to eat: A meal plan that works for the whole family

For some people, the hardest part of losing weight is deciding what—and how much—to eat. For others, it's the lack of variety or a seemingly never-ending battle with hunger. No matter what your challenge is, the meal plan in this chapter can help. It provides tasty, nutritious, portion- and calorie-controlled meals that are guaranteed to keep you satisfied, so you'll never feel deprived. Plus, it can be tailored for your entire family. Simply increase the portion sizes for anybody who isn't trying to lose weight (see "A special note for parents," page 19). That way, everyone can enjoy healthy meals.

Here's how it works: There are seven options provided for breakfast, lunch, and dinner, as well as a list of snacks. Unlike typical one-week meal plans, this plan allows you to mix and match meals and snacks, so it delivers flexibility, letting you enjoy different meal combinations daily for weeks on end.

You can also customize the options to suit your tastes by adding no-calorie flavor boosters like herbs and spices or a squirt of citrus. Love Asian food? Sprinkle five-spice powder on your pork tenderloin instead of adding sautéed apples and cinnamon. Looking for a Middle Eastern flair? Add the Moroccan spice blend called *ras el hanout* to your rotisserie chicken breast.

If you're a woman, simply choose one breakfast, lunch, dinner, and snack from the meals listed in this chapter. Men can follow the same program, but with two daily snacks to support their greater energy needs. That's all there is to it. No calorie counting or tracking grams of protein, carbohydrates, or fat. Just choose the meals that you like the best, and enjoy!

Breakfast

Skipping breakfast may sound tempting, but it only sets you up for hunger later in the day. Rely on these healthy 300-calorie options. They're packed with gradually digested protein to help you feel full until lunchtime.

▶ **Option 1**

Strawberry peanut butter oatmeal: Stir 1 teaspoon peanut butter into 1 cup cooked old-fashioned or steel-cut oatmeal. Top with ½ cup sliced strawberries.
1 cup nonfat milk.

▶ **Option 2**

Honey banana yogurt parfait: Stir 1 large pinch cinnamon into 1 cup plain nonfat Greek yogurt. Drizzle with 1 teaspoon honey. Top with 1 sliced banana and 1 tablespoon slivered almonds.

▶ **Option 3**

Cheesy egg sandwich: Fry or scramble 1 egg in 1 teaspoon olive oil. Serve on a toasted whole-wheat English muffin with sliced

www.health.harvard.edu   Lose Weight and Keep It Off

SPECIAL SECTION | What to eat: A meal plan that works for the whole family

tomato and 1 thin slice cheddar cheese.

▶ **Option 4**

Smoked salmon roll-up: Spread 1 tablespoon whipped cream cheese on an 8-inch whole-wheat tortilla. Top with 2 ounces smoked salmon and ¼ cup baby spinach. Roll up and slice in half.
Half a grapefruit.

▶ **Option 5**

Raspberry French toast: Dip 1 slice whole-wheat bread in 1 raw beaten egg. Cook in a sauté pan over medium heat in 1 teaspoon butter for 4 minutes, flipping midway. Top with ½ cup non-fat plain Greek yogurt and ½ cup raspberries.

▶ **Option 6**

Protein power plate: 1 hard-cooked egg, 10 walnut halves, and ¾ cup grapes.

▶ **Option 7**

Sweet cinnamon ricotta toast: Toast 2 slices whole-wheat bread. Top each slice with 1 tablespoon part-skim ricotta cheese and sprinkle with cinnamon.
1 pear.

Lunch

Instead of just grabbing whatever's easiest, go with these 400-calorie options. They have a perfect balance of protein, fiber, and complex carbs to keep you fueled all afternoon long.

▶ **Option 1**

Spicy roast chicken or turkey sandwich: Whisk ¼ teaspoon sriracha with 1 tablespoon light mayonnaise. Spread on 2 slices whole-wheat bread. Layer with 2 ounces roast chicken or turkey, 1 thin slice Swiss cheese, lettuce, and tomato.
1 sliced red bell pepper.

▶ **Option 2**

Black bean avocado burger: Layer 1 cooked black bean burger patty on 1 whole-wheat hamburger roll with ¼ sliced avocado, tomato slices, baby spinach, and 1 tablespoon barbeque sauce.
1 apple.

▶ **Option 3**

Tuna veggie pocket: Combine 3 ounces canned water-packed tuna, ¼ chopped cucumber, ¼ cup diced tomato, 1 tablespoon chopped red onion, 1 teaspoon chopped fresh basil, and 1 teaspoon each red wine vinegar and olive oil. Serve in a 6-inch whole-wheat pita.
1 orange.

▶ **Option 4**

Better-for-you Cobb salad: Toss together 2 cups shredded romaine lettuce, 1 diced hard-cooked egg, ½ cup diced tomato, ⅓ cup chickpeas, ¼ diced avocado, 3 chopped black olives, 1 tablespoon blue cheese crumbles, and 2 tablespoons balsamic vinaigrette.

▶ **Option 5**

Veggie burrito bowl: Sauté ½ cup sliced onions and ½ cup sliced green peppers in 1 teaspoon olive oil over medium heat for 5 minutes. Remove from heat and serve over 1 cup cooked brown rice with ½ cup warmed pinto beans, ½ cup diced tomato, 2 tablespoons salsa, and fresh cilantro to taste.

▶ **Option 6**

Open-faced veggie sandwich: Toast 2 slices whole-wheat bread. Top each slice with 2 tablespoons hummus, 2 basil leaves, and 1 slice roasted red pepper.
10 baby carrots.

▶ **Option 7**

Mediterranean salad: Toss together 2 cups baby spinach (or romaine lettuce), ½ cup rinsed and drained canned cannellini beans, 1 cup halved grape tomatoes, 2 tablespoons feta cheese crumbles, 1 tablespoon chopped walnuts, 2 teaspoons olive oil, and 1 tablespoon red wine vinegar.
10 small (1-inch) whole-wheat crackers.

 Dinner

Evening is the ideal time to fill in with foods you may not have had a chance to eat enough of during the day, like vegetables and whole grains. You'll find them all here in these satisfying 500-calorie dinners.

▶ **Option 1**

6 ounces grilled tuna steak.

What to eat: A meal plan that works for the whole family | **SPECIAL SECTION**

1 cup broccoli sautéed in 2 teaspoons peanut oil.

¾ cup cooked brown rice.

▶ Option 2

Spiced pork tenderloin: Season a 6-ounce boneless pork chop with one pinch each cinnamon and chili powder. Heat 2 teaspoons canola oil in a sauté pan over medium heat. Add pork and 1 sliced apple. Cook for 4 to 5 minutes, and flip pork chop and apple slices. Continue cooking 4 to 5 additional minutes, or until pork reaches an internal temperature of 145° F.

1 medium baked sweet potato.

▶ Option 3

Shrimp tostadas: Whisk together 2 tablespoons fresh lime juice with ¼ teaspoon chili powder. Add 10 large shelled, deveined shrimp and marinate for 10 minutes. Remove shrimp from marinade and broil or grill for 4 minutes, turning midway. Serve over 2 warmed 6-inch corn tortillas, topped with ½ cup shredded lettuce, ½ cup chopped tomato, ¼ cup tomato salsa, and fresh cilantro.

1 cup warmed black beans topped with 2 tablespoons shredded cheddar cheese.

▶ Option 4

4 ounces lean grilled sirloin steak.

1 medium baked potato with 1 tablespoon light sour cream.

1 cup romaine lettuce with 1 tablespoon Caesar dressing.

▶ Option 5

Pasta puttanesca with chicken: Heat 1 teaspoon olive oil in a sauté pan over medium heat. Add 2 ounces diced chicken tenders. Season with salt, pepper, and garlic powder. Cook for 6 minutes, stirring midway. Remove chicken from pan. Add ½ cup marinara sauce, 3 chopped black or kalamata olives, 1 teaspoon capers, and 1 pinch red pepper flakes. Cook over medium-low heat for 5 minutes. Remove from heat and toss with chicken and 1 cup cooked whole-wheat spaghetti. Top with 1 tablespoon grated Parmesan cheese.

8 asparagus spears sautéed in 1 teaspoon olive oil.

▶ Option 6

1 skinless rotisserie chicken breast.

1 cup Brussels sprouts sautéed in 2 teaspoons olive oil.

1 cup cooked quinoa tossed with ½ cup halved grape tomatoes and ½ teaspoon chopped fresh basil.

▶ Option 7

Vegetable stir-fry: Heat 1 tablespoon peanut oil in a large sauté pan or wok over high heat. Add 1 cup broccoli and ½ cup baby carrots and cook for 3 minutes. Add ½ cup shelled edamame, 1 tablespoon reduced-sodium soy sauce, 1 pinch red pepper flakes, and ¼ teaspoon each minced garlic and ginger. Cook for 1 additional minute. Remove from heat and serve over 1 cup cooked brown rice.

🍴 Snacks

Snacks are key for controlling hunger between meals. Each of these options provides a mix of protein, fiber, and healthy fat, and about 150 calories, to keep your appetite in check:

- 6-ounce container plain lowfat Greek yogurt topped with ½ cup raspberries
- 1 piece reduced-fat string cheese with 1 apple
- 3 tablespoons pumpkin or sunflower seeds
- 21 almonds, 12 walnut halves, or 45 pistachio nuts
- 4 cups air-popped microwave popcorn sprinkled with 1 tablespoon grated Parmesan
- 1 small banana with 2 teaspoons peanut, sunflower, or almond butter
- 2 1-inch cubes Brie cheese and ½ pear
- ¾ cup edamame
- 1 hard-cooked egg and 10 small (1-inch) whole-grain crackers
- ¾ cup 1% cottage cheese mixed with ½ cup blueberries
- 1 sliced red bell pepper with ¼ cup hummus
- 6-inch corn tortilla topped with ¼ cup mashed black beans, 1 tablespoon shredded cheddar cheese, and 1 tablespoon salsa
- One ounce of dark chocolate (at least 70% cacao). ♥

Tools that can help you lose weight

Losing weight requires all kinds of new habits, but sometimes it's difficult to know where to begin. That's especially true where eating habits are concerned. The truth is, optimal behaviors don't happen automatically. They require advance planning. When you wait until you're starving to eat, you don't always make the best choices. Think of the last time you walked in the door after a busy day and there was nothing healthy in the refrigerator. Maybe you picked up the phone to order a pizza. Or perhaps you grabbed a bag of potato chips that you could rip into immediately. Looking back, it's easy to see that these might not have been the best choices for weight loss, but when you're hungry, it can be hard to think clearly—especially if you're not prepared.

Instead, think about what would have happened if you'd had, say, a box of whole-wheat pasta and a jar of tomato sauce in the pantry, a package of frozen vegetables in the freezer, and a bag of baby carrots in the fridge. In less time than it would take to wait for take-out, you could have been snacking on the carrots while preparing a healthy meal, for a fraction of the calories of eating or ordering out.

If you're not much of a planner, don't worry. On the pages that follow, you'll find easy tips to help you stock your pantry with healthier foods, monitor your eating habits, and rearrange the food (and even the dishes) in your kitchen to reduce temptation.

Start by self-monitoring

If you've been gaining weight but aren't sure exactly why, it can be helpful to keep track of the changes. Perhaps the most common way is by using a scale (see "The scale: Friend or foe?" at right). But another very valuable tool is a food journal. Writing down what—and how much—you eat can help you become more aware of habits that are holding you back. It's so effective that one study found that people who recorded what they ate every day lost twice as much weight as people who didn't track their diets.

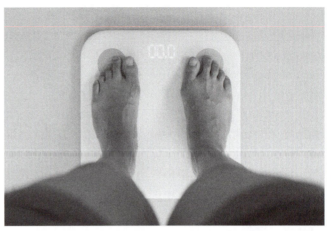

Weighing yourself several times a week can help keep you on track with weight loss, giving you an early warning sign when pounds are creeping on—and encouraging you when you're losing.

You can do it the old-fashioned way with a pen and paper, or you can go high-tech with a computer spreadsheet or smartphone app (see "The best smartphone apps for tracking food and exercise," page 25). Either way, be sure to write down every bite you take, both the good and the bad. This will help you pinpoint areas where you can improve. The more information you record, the better. For example, a more detailed diary that includes not just what you eat, but also how much, when, and where can be especially helpful. Some people also record their hunger levels before eating and their satisfaction levels afterward.

> ### The scale: Friend or foe?
>
> If you'll do anything to avoid stepping on the scale, you're hardly alone. Even so, you might want to give it another try. Research reveals that weighing yourself doesn't just help you lighten up, it can help you keep pounds off by letting you know if they are starting to sneak back on. And you don't need to weigh in every day. People who monitor themselves either daily or weekly are equally successful.

The best smartphone apps for tracking food and exercise

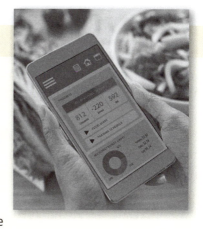

Your smartphone can make tracking diet and exercise easier than ever thanks to a growing number of weight-loss apps. Here are a few worth checking out.

Lose It. This app has a database of 32 million foods and exercises, and you can add your own custom foods and recipes. You can also use your smartphone camera to scan package bar codes and even log your food via photos. To keep you motivated, Lose It provides community support and allows you to sync with Apple Health and Google Fit. The paid version offers more perks, such as personal or group challenges for weight loss and exercise and connectivity with activity trackers and smart scales. Available for iPhone, Android, and desktop (free).

MyFitnessPal. As with Lose It, you can add your own favorite foods and recipes to MyFitnessPal's impressive database of 300 million entries, although there is a drawback to using entries generated by other users, as their accuracy is not guaranteed. It also contains a bar code scanner and a step tracker, and it connects with over 50 different fitness apps, smart scales, and fitness equipment. The exercise database allows you to track single activities or combine several activities into a custom workout. Available for iPhone and Android (free).

MyFoodDiary. This app tracks over 185,000 foods and 15 nutrients and lets you manually add new foods. It also analyzes your favorite recipes. Exercise-wise, MyFoodDiary calculates calories for more than 700 activities and provides motivational charts based on your personal exercise habits. There's a members-only discussion forum, and you can also link the app to a Fitbit. Available for iPhone and desktop ($9/month online membership).

MyNetDiary. Simply provide your target weight and MyNetDiary will create a personalized nutrition plan using its database of 800,000 verified foods and a Staple Food Catalog with more than 900 professionally chosen foods. It also tracks over 500 activities and exercises and allows you to create custom exercises. Contains a bar code scanner, and you can link to Apple Health, Apple Watch, Samsung Health, and Google Fit. Available for iPhone, Android, and desktop (free).

SparkPeople. This app's nutrition tracker includes a database of three million foods with a bar code scanner for fast entry. The fitness tracker includes more than 600 exercise demonstrations by certified trainers. Includes community message boards and challenges to boost motivation. Available for iPhone, Android, and desktop (free).

After you get started with your food journal, take a few minutes each day to figure out your typical pattern. Over time, you'll learn to identify circumstances where you were vulnerable to trigger foods—and learn to avoid those situations. For example, if you can't pass Dunkin' without stopping on your way to work, remap your route. If you can't resist the Cinnabon at the mall, shop somewhere else.

A food journal can also help you recognize habits that are standing in your way, such as eating when you weren't actually hungry, when you were feeling tired or depressed, or when you went back for seconds even though you were already full. Armed with this knowledge, you'll be able to develop strategies to avoid these common stumbling blocks in the future.

Reorganize your kitchen

You may not always be able to control what goes into the foods you eat outside of the house, but you can be in charge of those that you eat at home. Organizing your kitchen is one of the very best things you can do to jump-start your weight-loss efforts. To shape up your kitchen, try this six-step plan:

1. Hide snack foods. If you keep your salty or sugary snacks on the kitchen counter, find them a new home tucked away in the pantry. If they're not in your line of vision every time you enter the kitchen, you'll be less tempted to eat them. Researchers at Cornell University found that people who stored foods and beverages such as candy, cereal, and soda on their kitchen counters weighed 20 to 26 pounds more than people who kept these items out of sight. On the flip side, those who placed a bowl of fruit on the counter weighed 13 pounds less than people who didn't.

2. Revamp your refrigerator. Arrange the foods that you'd like to eat more of—such as fruits, vegetables, lean meats, eggs, hummus, low-fat milk, cottage cheese, and yogurt—at eye level in your fridge. That way, you'll be more likely to grab these first. At the same time, hide higher-fat items that you'd like to eat less of, such as cheese, out of sight in the deli drawer. Line your refrigerator doors with flavorful low-calorie condiments such as hot sauce, salsa, sriracha, ketchup, low-sodium soy sauce, and spicy mustard. Then, toss those that are high in fat, such as thick, gooey salad dressings (like ranch or thousand island) and tartar sauce. Finally, think about trading butter and cream cheese for lower-calorie whipped versions and swapping full-fat sour cream for a reduced-fat version.

3. Make your freezer friendlier. Your freezer can be a lifesaver when there's no time to shop for healthy food. Because frozen produce is flash frozen within hours of harvest, it's often nutritionally superior to fresh, which can sit on store shelves for days, losing nutrients all the while. Stock up on frozen vegetables for quick side dishes you can microwave in minutes. Think carrots, peas, broccoli, spinach, and edamame—you can even find interesting vegetable mixes, including some stir-fry blends. Any vegetable is fine, as long as it's free of cheese or buttery sauces.

4. Upgrade your pantry. Set aside some time to clean out and restock your pantry with these staples for quick and easy meals:

- **Quinoa, whole-wheat couscous, brown rice, and whole-wheat pasta.** Higher in fiber than white rice or noodles, these whole grains are gradually digested for prolonged energy and satiety.
- **Canned beans.** Whether they're black beans, pinto beans, or chickpeas, beans are a speedy way to add protein and fiber to salads, soups, and pasta.
- **Dried red lentils.** These offer up the same health benefits as beans, plus they cook in just 15 minutes.
- **Cold whole-grain cereal and rolled oats.** With these, you can make a nutrient-packed breakfast in minutes.
- **Air-popped or fat-free popcorn.** Everyone needs a crunchy snack sometimes. Make yours popcorn. You can eat five cups of air-popped popcorn for the same 150 calories you'd get from just 22 potato chips.
- **Canned tuna and salmon.** These lean proteins are a cinch to toss into salad or pasta on a busy weeknight.
- **Marinara sauce.** In addition to mixing with pasta, try spooning this sauce over grilled vegetables, baked potatoes, chicken breasts, or fish.
- **Vinegar.** Vinegar has been shown to smooth out spikes in post-meal blood sugar that can lead to hunger. Plus, it's nearly calorie-free.

5. Use smaller dishes. Bigger plates, glasses, and bowls almost always lead you to eat too much. The larger the dishes, the more food you fill them up with—and the more food you load onto your plate, the more you're likely to consume. Simply using a bowl that's 50% larger encourages you to eat 20% more food. To keep your portions in check, try replacing 12-inch dinner plates with 10-inch ones. Or else banish your dinner-sized plates to the back of your kitchen cabinets and move salad plates up front so they'll be the first thing you reach for when you set the table. Then take a close look at your bowls and serving dishes. Are they also oversized? If so, replace them with cereal bowls and invest in a few smaller bowls for soup and cereal. For snacks, try a small half-cup bowl or ramekin instead of a regular bowl. And don't forget to check out your drinking glasses. Many of these can hold 12 ounces of fluid or more. If you're using giant glasses for water or a big mug for unsweetened coffee or tea, go ahead and keep these up front. But if you're trying to cut down on sugary drinks, push large glasses and mugs to the back of the cabinet and move smaller juice-sized glasses and coffee cups to the front.

> **quicktip** | Spice up your food to add flavor without calories. Experiment with sweet-tasting herbs and spices like mint, cinnamon, allspice, clove, and nutmeg to add a sweet taste to foods. Try cinnamon instead of sugar to perk up your coffee, or mint to liven up iced tea.

> **fastfact** | Better food choices needn't cost a bundle. According to a Harvard study, eating right costs only about $1.50 more a day per person than an unhealthful diet.

6. Get the right gear. You don't have to go out and buy an entire kitchen's worth of new appliances to cook healthfully. However, there are a few basic gadgets that can help:

- **A kitchen scale.** Nutrition labels on many foods, such as dry pasta or cereal, list serving sizes in ounces, making them tricky to estimate. Weighing your portions can give you a good feeling for what a proper serving looks like.
- **Measuring spoons.** Use these for doling out high-calorie ingredients that can be difficult to eyeball, such as oil or peanut butter.
- **Dry measuring cups.** Try these instead of ladles or serving spoons for correctly sized portions every time.
- **Liquid measuring cups.** Use these for measuring tomato sauce, milk, or broth.
- **A spiralizer (or a vegetable peeler).** Lighten up your favorite pasta dish by eliminating the pasta altogether—instead, make veggie "noodles" from vegetables like zucchini, carrots, or beets.
- **A zester.** Citrus zest adds loads of flavor to fish, chicken, or pasta—and it's practically calorie-free. Zesters are also ideal for shredding cheese finely, so you'll use less of it.
- **Muffin tins.** Try these for perfectly portioned meat loaves or breakfast mini-frittatas.

Learn strategic shopping

The supermarket can be your best weight-loss ally—or your worst enemy. On one hand, it's filled with plenty of healthy whole foods that naturally tame hunger. On the other hand, it's also packed with high-calorie offenders (see "10 seemingly healthy foods to limit," above). If you're not careful, you can easily be coaxed into buying the less healthy choices, especially when many of these are positioned at eye level, where they're most visible.

When you visit the supermarket, start by shopping the perimeter. That's where you'll find plenty of whole foods such as fresh fruits and vegetables, whole-wheat bread, and low-fat dairy products, plus lean meat, chicken, and fish. Just keep in mind that store perimeters are increasingly being infiltrated by less healthful choices such as ice cream cases and displays of cookies and cakes. Even in the produce department, some salad kits include candied nuts and dressings high in sugar, so if a food isn't in its whole form, be sure to read the label carefully. Next, make your way toward the center aisles looking for foods with the shortest ingredient lists possible, such as whole grains, beans, canned tomatoes, whole-grain cereal, and frozen fruits and vegetables.

▶ 10 seemingly healthy foods to limit

Even foods with nutritious images and wholesome-sounding names can contain surprising amounts of sugar, processed carbohydrates, sodium, or fat. Be sure to read nutrition labels and watch portion sizes if you buy these foods:

- agave nectar
- bran muffins
- dried cranberries
- energy bars
- frozen yogurt
- fruit snacks
- granola
- pita chips
- trail mix
- turkey bacon.

Outsmarting the odds

Why do some people manage to stay slim even while living in an environment that promotes weight gain? Some, of course, are lucky to have a helpful complement of genes. Even if you don't, both physical activity and proper diet can often blunt a genetic tendency to be overweight. But there are also psychological factors at play.

Some of the tips in the previous chapter—for example, reorganizing your kitchen, using smaller dishes, and putting snack foods away—can play tricks on your mind that help you avoid the pitfalls of the famous "see-food diet" ("If I see food, I eat it") by reducing the amount of food in your line of sight. This chapter digs deeper by helping you reframe your mental attitude toward food.

Change your internal dialogue

Simply assuming that you have no power to change your weight can work against you. A study of 8,821 men and women found that those who felt they had no control over their weight were less likely to exercise and eat healthfully, and they were more likely to suffer from poor health as a result. What to do? Start by setting yourself a modest goal you know you can achieve, such as losing a few pounds, rather than aiming to reverse decades of weight gain in six months. Each mini-goal you achieve reinforces the new habits you're learning and also increases your confidence.

Changing your beliefs about food can even affect the hunger-regulating hormones your body secretes. Yale University researchers put this theory to the test by offering volunteers a 380-calorie milkshake on two separate occasions. Even though the researchers knew that all of the milkshakes contained the same amount of calories, they told the volunteers that they were drinking a 620-calorie "indulgent" milkshake on one occasion, and then advised them that they were sipping a 140-calorie "sensible" milkshake on the other.

After each milkshake, the researchers measured the volunteers' ghrelin levels. Amazingly, when the volunteers thought they were drinking the indulgent milkshake, their levels of ghrelin (the hunger-boosting hormone) took a nosedive afterward. However, when they believed they were drinking the sensible milkshake, their ghrelin levels barely budged, providing them with little satisfaction.

The take-home message isn't that you should lie to yourself and pretend that steamed broccoli is an indulgent dessert (although it can taste delicious in a light lemon-caper sauce). Rather, boost your satisfaction with simple techniques like adding spices to foods and paying more attention to the textures and flavors in your meals (see "Slow down—and try mindful eating," page 31).

Control comfort eating

There's a reason people reach for foods like French fries or cookies when they're feeling down. It makes them feel better. "We know that there are parts of the brain that are rewarded from eating high-fat or high-sugar foods. And over a decade of psychological research tells us that any behavior that is rewarded is likely to be repeated," says Stephanie Sogg, an assistant professor in the Department of Psychiatry at Harvard Medical School. "So, if you eat for comfort and you find that it works, you're naturally going to do it again." The trouble is, comfort eating—also known as emotional or stress eating—only works temporarily. Worse, it causes longer-term distress if it brings about weight gain.

The first step: Begin by finding out why you need comfort food. Does it calm you down, cheer you up, compensate you for a tough day, or some combination? Simply recognizing these thought patterns can make it easier to resist giving in. It's also helpful to realize the longer-term implications. "Eating never solves the problem that made you upset," says

Try cognitive behavioral therapy

It's all too common a sequence: you have a fight with your partner, and the next thing you know you're drowning your sorrows in a chocolate bar. But what we often don't realize is that somewhere in between the argument and the chocolate bar, there's a thought that tells us that eating sweets will make us feel better.

Cognitive behavioral therapy, or CBT, is a form of personalized psychological therapy that encourages you to discover and expose negative and unproductive ways of thinking (and therefore acting)—such as grabbing a chocolate bar when you're stressed—and teaches you to replace these patterns with more helpful ones. In CBT for obesity, therapists help their patients identify and change the sabotaging thoughts that perpetuate overeating and weight gain (as well as others related to personal issues, such as appearance, self-confidence, and quality of friendships).

"We can't stop people from feeling stressed, angry, or sad, but what we can do is help them with what they say to themselves that causes them to eat and help them come up with a different response, so that next time the behavior or action will be more productive," says Deborah Beck Busis, program director for the Beck Institute for Cognitive Behavior Therapy, which offers CBT for weight management. Then, next time you have a run-in with your partner, you might say to yourself, "Sure, I'm really upset and I hate feeling this way, but if I eat to soothe myself, I'll feel upset about the fight *and* about my weight, too. Instead, I'll go for a walk so I can calm down and feel better."

Deborah Beck Busis, program director for the Beck Institute for Cognitive Behavior Therapy outside Philadelphia. "It ultimately just makes the situation worse because it creates even more problems by jeopardizing weight loss, reinforcing bad habits, and making you feel guilty."

The best way to learn your triggers for comfort eating is to keep a food diary that records not only what and how much you ate, but also how you felt at the time (see "Start by self-monitoring," page 24). Once you learn to recognize a pattern, you can develop a strategy to break it. For instance, if you often eat because you think you deserve it after a tough day, "remember that you also deserve to lose weight, feel healthy, and be proud of yourself," says Busis. If you eat because of stress, learn to dial back that stress (see "Lower your stress level," page 35).

The second step: Distract yourself from the lure of comfort foods. The best distractions are things that take only about five minutes—just long enough to help you switch gears, but not so long they're impractical. Following are some ideas for switching gears:

- Go for a five-minute walk.
- Take a hot shower or bath.
- Sit outside in the sunshine.
- Put on your favorite music and dance around the house.
- Listen to your favorite podcast.
- Call your best friend to chat.

The more ways you can think of to distract yourself, the easier it will become over time to resist the siren call of comfort food. Instead, resisting will become your new habit. If you can't do this on your own, you might try cognitive behavioral therapy (see box at left).

Learn to tell hunger from cravings

"Have some cake, it's a celebration!" "Don't eat because dinner's in an hour." "Hurry up and eat now because lunchtime will be over soon." From the time we're toddlers, we're taught to ignore our feelings of hunger and fullness. Researchers have found that between ages 3 and 5, we start paying more attention to behavioral cues and less attention to hunger signals from our bodies. So, it's no wonder many of us have difficulty distinguishing between genuine hunger and cravings.

The difference? Physical hunger is an emptiness you feel in the pit of your stomach. A craving is more likely to be a sense of discomfort or agitation in your mouth or your head. If you're not sure which one you're feeling, try one of these strategies:

- **Take the tofu test.** When you're truly hungry, you'll eat just about anything. Ask yourself, "Would I be willing to eat tofu, celery, or carrots?" If the answer is yes, it's likely hunger. Cravings, by contrast, are generally for a particular food or drink—especially a comfort food. Chocolate, anyone?
- **Rank it.** Try to rate your hunger versus fullness on a scale of 0 (ravenous) to 10 (stuffed). If you feel the urge to eat, but you're not hungry—say, at neutral (5)

or even toward the direction of full—then it's likely a craving, especially if you're fixating on some special food.

- **Wait it out.** Most cravings go away in 15 or 20 minutes. Hunger doesn't. It only gets stronger.

When you have cravings, the question then becomes how to fight back. Waiting it out is good, but often hard to do. Some of the strategies listed earlier for distracting yourself are good ways to fight a craving (see "Control comfort eating," page 28). Here are some others:

- Brush your teeth; the mint flavor of the toothpaste can often help quell a craving.
- What you perceive as a desire for food is often thirst. Drink a glass of water, then reassess whether you still need to eat.
- Distance yourself physically from the food. If you can see or smell tempting food, it's harder to resist.

If you still can't stop thinking about a food after 15 minutes, go ahead and give yourself permission to eat a small, preplanned portion. The good news is that the more often you manage to resist cravings, the less intense and the less frequent they become.

Sidestep temptation

As you know all too well, we're surrounded by tempting foods. But the pizza parties after your kids' soccer game or the donut boxes at office staff meetings aren't going to disappear. The trick is to develop a strategy to deal with them, so they don't get the better of you.

The first step: Don't allow yourself to become overly hungry. Get in the habit of regularly ranking your feelings of hunger and fullness throughout the day using a scale of 0 (ravenous) to 10 (stuffed). When you start to feel the level approaching that slightly hungry stage (say, around 3 to 4), if it's not close to mealtime, then reach for a healthy snack. To make sure that you're not grabbing the first thing that you can get your hands on—which is all too often a sweet or salty load of processed carbs—plan healthy portion-controlled snacks in advance and carry them with you. Good choices include an apple and a piece of string cheese or a 1-ounce baggie of nuts.

The second step: Whenever possible, create a plan to deal with temptation ahead of time. If you know that your co-worker is going to bring in brownies on Friday, Busis recommends writing down a response in advance on a note card that you can read in the morning, such as "My body doesn't know or care what everyone else is eating. It only knows what I eat, so if I do eat that brownie, it will sabotage my weight-loss goals. Instead, I'm going to wait and eat a special portion-controlled treat that I've planned for tonight." Then, rather than hanging out in the break room where the brownies are, sit at your desk and return a few phone calls instead.

If the temptation comes unexpectedly, try again to remember your larger goals. Maybe you want to lose weight to reduce your blood pressure, or help get your blood sugar under control, or look better for an upcoming event.

Don't go to extremes

Nothing seems more unfair than feeling like you can't eat what everyone else is eating. "It stinks that some people can eat whatever they want, but if you want to lose weight, you have to modify your eating," says Sogg. "The key is to do it in a moderate way." Experts agree: extreme deprivation always backfires. It's simply a matter of time.

One way to keep from feeling deprived is to use the techniques in "Sidestep temptation" (at left). Another is to allow yourself to eat the foods you love, but less of them. So, if you know you love the Boston cream pie at your favorite restaurant, ask for two forks and share the dessert with your dinner companion. The first few bites invariably deliver the most satisfaction, so if you savor them, you may feel just as happy with half a slice as with a whole one (see "Slow down—and try mindful eating," page 31).

Or, if you know you'll never be able to eat just half a cup of ice cream, go ahead and have a whole cup. Just make sure that if you're at home, you measure the ice cream out into a bowl rather than eating it directly from the container, or else you might end up eating the whole pint. "Moderation is difficult," says Sogg. "It's a skill you have to work at, but it works better than all or nothing."

Help for binge eating disorder

People who frequently overeat may have binge eating disorder, the most common eating disorder in the United States. Roughly 3% of Americans have this condition, which means that they frequently consume extremely large quantities of food in one sitting—and feel out of control while doing so. Other hallmarks of the condition include eating quickly, often to the point of discomfort; frequently eating alone; hoarding food and hiding empty food containers; and feeling depressed, disgusted, or upset about their uncontrollable eating.

Fewer than half the people who have binge eating disorder seek treatment for the problem, but psychotherapy—particularly cognitive behavioral therapy—can help (see "Try cognitive behavioral therapy," page 29).

With moderation, you may not lose weight as fast as you would on an extreme diet, but you'll probably have more success keeping off what you do lose and sticking with your plan over time.

Slow down—and try mindful eating

When was the last time you enjoyed a quiet, peaceful meal without interruption? If you can't remember, you're hardly alone. These days, eating a leisurely meal is a rare luxury. Sadly, for many people, eating on the run has become the norm. They gobble down meals while they text their friends, catch up on their favorite TV shows, or check to see who's posting on Twitter and Facebook. Yet research reveals that the very act of eating in a hurry may contribute to overweight and obesity.

Here's how. As you eat and drink, your stomach fills, activating stretch receptors in your stomach. These receptors send satiety messages to your brain via the vagus nerve, which connects the brain to the stomach. Then, as food enters your small intestine, appetite hormones are released, sending additional fullness messages to your brain. This process doesn't happen immediately, though. It can take 20 minutes—or longer—for your brain to realize it's time to put down your fork. Eating too quickly doesn't allow this intricate system sufficient time to work, making it easy to overeat without even realizing it.

There's another downside to distracted eating that has nothing to do with speed. Eating while you're busy doing other things robs you of the opportunity to fully enjoy your food, so you may not feel completely satisfied—and may keep on eating in an attempt to gain satisfaction.

Enter mindful eating. Mindful eating is the act of fully focusing on your food as you eat. It encourages you to pay closer attention to the tastes, smells, and textures of your food as well as your body's hunger and satiety cues. As basic as it sounds, this practice is surprisingly powerful. In one small study, 10 obese volunteers enrolled in weekly mindful eating classes that focused on listening to their feelings of hunger and fullness. They also paid close attention to their cravings and emotions. Not only did the participants drop an average of 9 pounds by the end of the three-month program, but they also reported less hunger, stress, anxiety, depression, and binge eating (see "Help for binge eating disorder," above left).

In addition to savoring the flavors and aromas of your food, the following techniques can help you attain more mindful eating:

- Eat only at the kitchen or dining room table to minimize distractions.
- Create a calm, beautiful space for eating. A cluttered table does not create the sense of inner tranquility you need in order to cultivate a peaceful mindset.
- At the beginning of your meal, set a timer for 20 minutes. Then pace yourself to make your meal last until the timer goes off.
- Let incoming phone calls go to voicemail or the answering machine.
- Put away all computers, phones, and reading materials, so you can concentrate on your food.
- Turn off the television, another source of distraction.
- Think only about the bite of food you're actually eating at that moment. It's all too easy to think ahead to the next bite without focusing on the food that's actually in your mouth.
- Put your fork down between bites.
- Chew each mouthful 30 times.
- Before you help yourself to seconds or dessert, ask yourself if you're really hungry (see "Learn to tell hunger from cravings," page 29).

The exercise equation

"Diet and exercise"—the words have become permanently linked in discussions not only of weight management, but of health in general, and for good reason. Regular physical activity can help you live longer by decreasing your risk of heart disease, diabetes, and certain cancers. It also keeps your bones strong, eases joint pain, tunes up immune function, improves your sleep, protects mental health, and boosts your mood. And though exercise takes a backseat to diet in the area of weight loss, it still plays an important role in weight management—especially when it comes to maintaining weight loss.

Why moving matters

First, the bad news. There are multiple reasons why exercise is not as effective as diet for weight loss. For starters, a good exercise session is likely to make you hungry, so don't be surprised if you eat back a lot of the calories you just burned. Moreover, you have to work much harder than you might think to work off weight. Think about it this way: for the average 150-pound person, an hour of walking at 3 mph burns 250 calories. If you reward yourself afterward with a chocolate chip Clif bar, you'll replace those calories in a matter of minutes.

That said, you can't ignore exercise either, if you want to shed weight and keep it off. Exercise does burn calories, even if it doesn't work off as many as you might hope. Surprisingly, even small movements like fidgeting make a difference (see "That's NEAT!" on page 33). Equally important, regular exercise boosts your metabolic rate, even when you're not exercising. This is crucial,

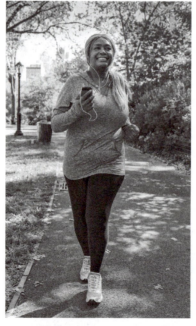

Exercise helps you burn calories. Even after you finish your workout, it boosts your metabolism for a while.

since your metabolism slows as you shed pounds. Exercise can keep your rate higher, helping to battle those frustrating plateaus. The harder you work out, the longer it will last. In a study published in *Medicine and Science in Sports and Exercise*, 45 minutes of vigorous exercise boosted metabolism for 14 hours afterward in 10 young men.

Aerobic exercise, such as walking or running, plays an obvious role in calorie burn. But strength training also contributes, for a simple reason. Most fat cells store calories, but they don't burn them. Muscle cells do. As you age, you lose muscle mass. And if you're trying to lose weight solely by cutting calories, you're likely losing even more muscle. According to one study, 27% of the weight lost by dieting alone comes from muscle. Combining dieting with cardio exercise cuts muscle loss in half—but when you combine dieting with strength training, all the pounds lost come from fat.

For all the emphasis on calorie burn, however, new research indicates that physical activity helps regulate weight in ways that go well beyond energy expenditure. For example, a combination of aerobic exercise and strength training boosts levels of a hormone-like substance called irisin, which is generated in skeletal muscles and travels through the bloodstream to fat tissue and other organs. Irisin nudges the composition of fat tissue in a healthier direction by turning some of your white fat cells (which are mainly storage depots for calories) into beige cells (which resemble energy-burning, heat-producing brown cells). Irisin levels naturally decline with age, so exercise is an important way of keeping up levels in older adults. High levels of irisin are associated with greater muscle mass and strength, as well as greater insulin sensitivity—an important factor for anyone with diabetes. By contrast, low levels correlate with obesity and insulin resistance.

Exercise also enhances your gut bacteria, which may seem unrelated to weight unless you think back to the explanation under "Gut instinct" on page 5. In one study, researchers analyzed gut bacteria in 40 professional rugby players in preseason training and two groups of less active men, 23 whose weight fell into the healthy range and another 23 who were either overweight or obese. The rugby players had substantially more diverse gut bacteria than either of the other groups. Of particular interest, they had higher levels of the bacterium *Akkermansia muciniphila*, which is believed to be associated with lower levels of obesity and related metabolic disorders.

Other intriguing research, this time in mice, suggests that exercise makes your brain more responsive to leptin, the hormone that tells you when you have enough energy on board. Normally when you lose weight, leptin levels fall, prompting you to eat more and put weight back on. Exercise helps counter that response. Plus, vigorous exercise like running may actually help suppress appetite. When nine female walkers and 10 runners exercised for 60 minutes and then had a meal, the walkers ate back all of the calories they burned off and a few extra, according to a study in the *Journal of Obesity*. The runners, by contrast, still had a deficit of nearly 200 calories even after eating.

Finally, exercise relieves stress and improves your mood, helping to dial back emotional eating. In a study in *The American Journal of Clinical Nutrition*, researchers followed 421 people for a year and rated them every three months on measures such as cravings, eating restraint, and exercise. The volunteers who were the least active reported the most food cravings and were roughly two to four times more likely to gain weight than those who were moderately active.

That's NEAT!

While regular exercise is important for your general health, even very small amounts of energy expenditure, such as standing instead of sitting, can add up when it comes to weight loss. So do small actions, such

▶ 15 ways to burn 150 calories

There are many ways to burn calories—through both formal exercise and everyday activity. In each of the following examples, 150 calories is an estimate; the precise amount will vary from person to person.

1. Dance for 30 minutes.
2. Bicycle four miles in 15 minutes or five miles in 30 minutes.
3. Wash and wax your car for 45 to 60 minutes.
4. Play volleyball for 45 minutes.
5. Garden for 30 to 45 minutes.
6. Push a stroller for 1.5 miles in 30 minutes.
7. Run 1.5 miles in 15 minutes.
8. Rake leaves for 30 minutes.
9. Walk two miles in 30 minutes.
10. Do water aerobics for 30 minutes.
11. Swim laps for 20 minutes.
12. Wash your windows or floors for 45 to 60 minutes.
13. Play basketball for 15 to 20 minutes.
14. Jump rope for 15 minutes.
15. Climb stairs for 15 minutes.

as fidgeting or tapping your foot while you sit at your desk. In fact, such habits may represent one factor that separates lean people from their heavier counterparts.

This type of movement, called non-exercise activity thermogenesis, or NEAT, is so powerful that it can burn hundreds of extra calories a day. Fidgeting alone kicks up calorie burn by roughly 5%. But if you stand up and move around, you'll do even better. A man who works as a cashier on his feet all day and plays the guitar in his free time can burn 1,000 calories more per day than a man of the same size who sits in front of a computer at work and watches TV at night—even if neither one does any formal kind of exercise. Someone with a physically strenuous job can burn up to 2,000 calories more per day than a sedentary desk jockey.

Even if you're not normally a NEAT type, you can train yourself to boost this kind of activity. Pace around your home or office while you talk on the phone. Walk down the hall to talk to a co-worker instead of emailing or phoning. Or be a little less efficient when you're cleaning the house by alternating tasks on different floors, so you have to go up and down stairs more often. Anything will help.

Getting started

Some 60% of American adults don't meet government recommendations for physical activity, and 25% aren't physically active at all. For many people, the very idea of exercise sounds daunting. But it doesn't have to be. If you haven't been active, walking is often a good option to begin with, because all you really need is a good pair of shoes. Harvard Medical School has a number of Special Health Reports dedicated to exercise programs for beginners—including *Starting to Exercise, Walking for Health, A Beginner's Guide to Running, Gentle Core Exercises*, and *Strength and Power Training for All Ages* (see "Resources," page 53, for ordering information). A number of other Special Health Reports are geared to those who are more advanced. *Note:* If you have not been active recently, if you have injuries, or if you have a chronic health condition, such as obesity, heart disease, or diabetes, speak with your physician before you start any new physical activity program. He or she may want to suggest modifications for your safety. If you're uncertain whether you should talk with a doctor, consult the Get Active Questionnaire from the Canadian Society for Exercise Physiology (www.health.harvard.edu/GAQ).

Assuming you're fit and active, how much exercise is enough? Any amount is beneficial. But for modest weight loss, the American College of Sports Medicine (ACSM) recommends 150 to 250 minutes per week of moderate aerobic activity, such as brisk walking. Benefits are greater at the higher end of that range, but 30 minutes of daily exercise puts you well in the zone. For clinically significant weight loss, the ACSM recommends ratcheting up to more than 250 minutes a week. Don't be afraid to mix it up. For other moderate-intensity activities, you might play doubles tennis, mow the lawn, ride a bicycle on flat ground, or do water aerobics. For more ideas, see "15 ways to burn 150 calories" on page 33.

In addition to aerobic activity, the ACSM recommends two weekly strength training workouts that target all of your major muscle groups, including your arms, shoulders, legs, hips, abdomen, and chest, to help maintain calorie-burning muscle tissue. Lifting weights, working out with resistance bands or tubes, using weight machines, or such activities as heavy gardening all count. Be sure to allow 48 hours between strength sessions to give your muscles time to recover.

Staying motivated

It happens to everyone on occasion: you tossed and turned all night, so you're too exhausted to lace up your walking shoes the next morning. Or maybe you had a rough day at the office and you just want to go home and flop on the couch. There are countless reasons why you might be too tired to exercise. But here's why you should ignore them and go to the gym anyway: it turns out that exercise can actually boost your energy. It increases the amount of oxygen and nutrients that are delivered to your tissues, nudges up levels of energy-producing mitochondria in your cells, and improves your sleep. Moreover, it just makes you feel better by increasing your blood levels of endorphins—the "feel-good" chemicals that are often credited for the "runner's high."

Some people find that wearable fitness trackers—such as Fitbit and Garmin—help keep them motivated. But you don't have to go high-tech. People who use a pedometer also tend to log more physical activity.

Here are some tricks requiring no equipment at all to help keep your momentum up:

- **Mark exercise on the calendar.** It can be hard to find time to exercise. Keep your workouts on track by scheduling them like other appointments.
- **Recruit a workout buddy.** Having a friend work out with you makes it harder to skip sessions and makes working out more fun, too.
- **Lay out your exercise clothes (or pack your gym bag) the night before.** Seeing your workout gear all ready to go makes it harder to make excuses.
- **Sign up for a class.** If you reserve a space, you'll be less likely to cancel.
- **Start with 10 minutes.** Lack of time is a common excuse for not exercising, but almost anyone can find 10 minutes. Even a light workout is better than none at all. Chances are once you get going, you'll be inspired to do more.

Other lifestyle changes that help shed pounds

Once you decide to take off weight, it's only natural to want to reach your goal as quickly as possible. But keep in mind that those pounds took years to sneak up on you, even though it sometimes seems like they magically appeared overnight. In reality, most people gain only about a pound a year. Over the decades, that can slowly snowball into 20, 30, or 40 pounds or more. And while it's easy to blame those gains on a less-than-perfect diet, it's important to keep in mind that other lifestyle factors play a profound role in weight gain as well.

This chapter delves into five of the top lifestyle reasons for weight gain—and how you can fight them.

Lower your stress level

Have you ever wondered why you crave foods like ice cream or cupcakes when you're stressed? The reason isn't just that they're decadent and delicious. There are biological mechanisms at play, too. Foods that contain large amounts of fat and sugar can genuinely make you feel better when you're feeling down or harried.

How does that happen? When a stressful event is brief—such as a traffic jam or a fight with your spouse or partner—it usually inhibits your appetite, at least for the short term. But when stress becomes chronic—for example, if you spend every day in a tense office environment or care for a sick parent or child—your adrenal glands secrete the hormone cortisol, which stimulates appetite and makes you crave less-than-healthy, fatty, sugary foods. Research has found that these foods soothe stress centers in the brain. Some people may be particularly sensitive to the calming effect of these foods, as research has shown that people who produce larger amounts of cortisol when they're tense may be more likely to reach for snacks when they're under pressure.

At the same time, stress often goes hand in hand with anxiety and depression, both of which can trigger emotional eating. If emotional eating happens occasionally, it's not much of an issue. But if you usually eat when you're tense, anxious, or depressed, try these strategies to decompress:

Take some deep breaths. Your breathing can have a direct physiological effect on your body. Slow, rhythmic breathing activates your parasympathetic nervous system, which promotes a relaxed state. Your heart rate slows, and hormones that promote feelings of calm and social bonding increase. The opposite happens with fast, superficial breathing patterns. Heart rate increases, and stress hormones are released.

Get moving. Exercise naturally releases brain chemicals known as endorphins that calm and relax you. Try a brisk 20-minute walk around your neighborhood—or the mall, if your area isn't walkable. Or, try out an online fitness or dance video from a site such as Fitness Blender (www.fitnessblender.com) or Popsugar Fitness (www.popsugar.com/Class-Fitsugar).

Phone a friend. Social support has been shown to reduce stress. Instead of going it alone, reach out to a pal or loved one next time you're feeling overwhelmed.

Unplug. Checking your email all day long is a sneaky source of stress. One study found that when individuals limited the number of times they opened their email to three times a day, they reported less stress and a greater sense of well-being than when they continuously checked their inboxes.

Write it down. Jot down your feelings without worrying about grammar or punctuation. This practice, known as expressive writing, has been shown to improve psychological, social, and physical health.

> **fast fact** | A 2016 study in the *Journal of Clinical Sleep Medicine* found that people who ate more saturated fat slept less soundly and awakened more frequently. On the flip side, those who ate more fiber experienced more restorative deep slow-wave sleep.

Avoid the TV trap

Increased TV time has been linked to greater body weight. A large trial that was part of the long-running Nurses' Health Study followed more than 50,000 women for six years and found that for every two hours a day that a woman spent watching TV, her risk of obesity increased by 23% and her odds of developing diabetes climbed by 14%. Part of the problem is that when people watch TV, they are completely sedentary, instead of participating in other activities that require more energy. In fact, watching TV burns only slightly more calories than sleeping, and less than other sedentary activities such as reading. Food advertisements may also play a significant role, tempting you to go to the kitchen to hunt for a snack.

In addition to reducing screen time over all, try these tips to mitigate the effects of the time you do spend in front of the TV:

- Stand up during commercials and move around.
- Buy a minicycle that you can put in front of your chair to pedal while watching.
- Stretch during the show.
- Record your favorite shows and watch them later, so you can fast-forward through the tempting food commercials—and reduce total screen time.

Even better, forgo the show and buy an active video game that forces you to move. Note that sedentary time in front of the computer can be just as problematic as TV time. The more absorbed you are in your work or entertainment, the easier it is to eat mindlessly.

Get enough sleep

An emerging body of research reveals that the less you sleep, the more likely you are to put on excess weight. One trial followed 83,377 men and women for seven-and-a-half years. The researchers found that those who were not initially obese but slumbered fewer than five hours a night were 40% more likely to develop obesity by the study's end compared with those who slept for seven to eight hours a night.

Too little shut-eye seems to promote weight gain in several ways (see Figure 2, below). For starters, lack of sufficient sleep has been shown to slow metabolism, so you burn fewer calories. Plus, the resulting fatigue can make you less motivated to be up and about the next day, and more likely to spend the day sitting or lounging around. At the same time, sleep deprivation disrupts hormones that control hunger and appetite, such as leptin and ghrelin, which may be why research shows that a lack of sleep can encourage you to eat

Figure 2: How sleep loss may lead to weight gain

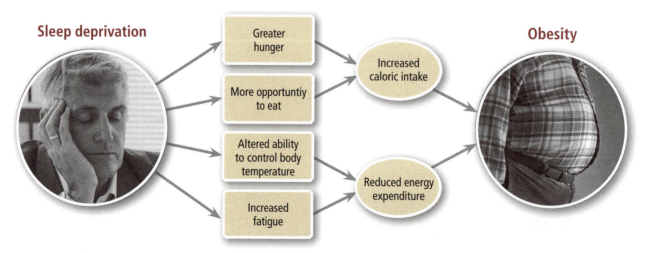

Staying up too late at night means you'll have more opportunities to eat, but that's not the only problem. Sleep deprivation can alter your body's metabolism, slowing it down and making you feel hungrier. You will also feel more tired during the day, which means you're less likely to exercise. To boost your energy, you'll be more apt to reach for some hassle-free comfort foods, such as a donut or bag of potato chips, which quickly pack on the pounds.

300 to 550 extra calories a day—in particular, quickly digested carbs, which give you short energy spurts but don't ultimately alleviate your fatigue.

If you'd like a better night's sleep, try these tips from the National Sleep Foundation:

- **Stay active.** Exercise helps regulate your body clock, particularly when done during daylight hours.
- **Make sleep a priority.** Don't let sleep be the thing you do only after everything else is done. Schedule it like any other activity.
- **Stay on schedule.** Going to sleep at the same time every night helps your body know when it's time to feel sleepy. People with a regular sleep schedule are 3.5 times more likely to say they feel well rested on any given weekday.
- **Practice good sleep hygiene.** Use your bed only for sleeping or sex. Don't use electronic devices within two hours of your bedtime, as the blue light they emit keeps you wakeful. Keep your room as dark and quiet as possible. And if you don't fall asleep in 20 to 30 minutes, get up and go to another room to read or do something calming until you feel sleepy.

Given that lack of sleep has also been found to affect the risk for chronic diseases such as diabetes, heart disease, and Alzheimer's, maintaining a regular sleep schedule is a smart move.

Eat earlier in the day

A long-held axiom of dieting maintains that "a calorie is a calorie is a calorie." If that were strictly true, it wouldn't matter when you eat. But research is increasingly showing that it's better to eat earlier in the day than to pack in the bulk of your calories later.

In part, this has to do with the types of food you're likely to eat as the day advances. If you come home from work ravenous, you're more likely to wolf down sweet or salty snacks before dinner. Late-night snacks can be even more insidious, as many people eat excess calories to soothe cravings. Perhaps that's why studies show that people who consume more of their calories at night tend to be heavier and have more difficulty shedding unwanted pounds.

However, metabolic factors may also play a role. Health experts are now learning that your metabolism has its own circadian rhythm. Given that food is essentially fuel for your muscles and metabolism, when you eat may play a surprising role in how much you weigh. In one study, dieting women who ate lunch after 3 p.m. lost less weight than those who lunched earlier, even though both groups had similar diets and calorie intake.

While researchers aren't sure exactly why eating later leads to greater weight gain, a Harvard Medical School study found that when people ate a meal in the evening, the thermic effect of their food (the amount of energy it takes to digest that food) was an astounding 44% lower than when they ate the identical meal in the morning. In other words, your body's natural rhythms determine when you burn the most and the fewest calories. Other researchers suspect that eating late in the day or at night may hinder the body's ability to use insulin and glucose efficiently, promoting fat storage.

Recruit supportive friends

The company you keep could affect your body weight. In one analysis of data from the long-running Framingham Heart Study, researchers calculated that a normal-weight person had a 2% chance per year of developing obesity—but those odds increased by half a percentage point for every social contact he or she had who was obese. Translated into real-life terms, that means that having four severely overweight friends would double your chances of developing obesity. On the flip side, research has found that having leaner friends is linked to lower body weight.

Why this happens isn't clear, although one likely explanation is that your view of what is normal to eat changes depending on what you see your friends and loved ones eating. Another reason may be behavioral. For example, having friends who spend more time working out or playing sports may inspire you to be more active as well.

This doesn't mean that you should jettison your friends. But it does mean that you need to be aware of the influence other people's habits can have on you. To counteract this, try forming alliances with friends and family members who will help support you in your weight-loss endeavor—especially if they're trying to lose weight, too.

Weight-loss programs and diets

A staggering 161 million Americans are on a diet, spending a collective $72 billion annually in their quest to achieve a healthy body weight. To reach their goals, some people turn to the latest popular diets. Others enroll in a commercial plan, such as Weight Watchers or Jenny Craig; or sign up for diet meals to be delivered to their doorsteps; or join an online program.

Which of these approaches can *really* help you lose weight? The answer is any one that offers a diet you can happily stick with for the long haul. Just make sure that any program you pick is balanced in nutrients, offers plenty of great-tasting and healthy choices, and does not require an extensive or expensive list of groceries or supplements.

To help you find the tools you need to reach your goal, this chapter gives a quick overview of the most popular commercial weight-loss plans, home meal delivery services, online programs, and weight-loss regimens.

Commercial programs

If you're the type of person who thrives on motivation and support, a commercial diet program might be worth looking into. These programs hold regular in-person or virtual meetings to provide direction, guidance, and encouragement. Many also supply exercise advice as well as online tools for tracking your weight and food intake, and several have programs specifically designed for people with diabetes. Keep in mind that weight loss may be modest: a 2017 analysis of published research studies found that 57% of people who start a commercial program lose less than 5% of their starting weight.

While purchasing the prepared foods offered by some of these programs can boost your success, it's not the main factor that makes them so effective. In one study, researchers concluded that the *structure* these programs provide in the form of regular calorie-controlled meals is likely the key to their success. Having other people around you who are striving for the same goal can help, too. One study found that when people invited someone to join a weight-loss program with them, those who had a successful partner lost roughly 10% of their body weight in 18 months—roughly double the amount lost by people who joined solo or whose partner didn't drop any weight.

There are several factors you should consider when looking for commercial programs. Does the program offer balanced food and exercise choices? What are the credentials of the people who are running the program?

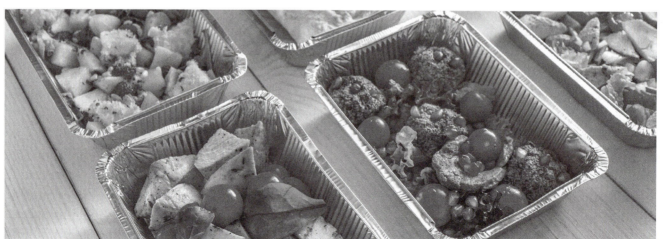

Meal delivery programs can take the guesswork out of weight loss by providing calorie- and portion-controlled meals.

Is there a maintenance program? How much weight, on average, do clients regain over the long term? Is the program offered in person or online? Are you required to buy special foods? What are the total costs, including membership, weekly fees, counseling, and any special foods? Finally, check with your doctor before starting one of these programs, because some of them—though not the ones listed here—are very restrictive and use supplements, weight-loss medications, or both.

Here are two examples of popular commercial programs and what you can expect from them:

WW (Weight Watchers). WW has 4.2 million subscribers worldwide and more than five decades of experience. Two trials showed that people who attended meetings regularly lost about 5% of their body weight within three to six months. Meetings are led by members who have successfully lost weight and kept it off.

In 2020, the company introduced its new MyWW program, which encourages physical activity plus a healthy diet, using a system called SmartPoints that allocates a point value to every food based on calories and nutrition. Under this system, any food is allowed, but some foods—including more than 300 ZeroPoint foods—are more desirable than others. SmartPoints steer members toward lean protein, fruits, and vegetables, and away from saturated fat and sugar. ZeroPoint foods pose low risk of overeating.

After a comprehensive assessment of food preferences, activity level, lifestyle, and approach to weight loss, members are matched to one of three plans, each with a different balance of ZeroPoint foods and SmartPoints. Members also earn FitPoints for engaging in physical activity, which can be swapped for SmartPoints. The plan is offered at three different levels: digital, digital plus meetings, or digital with personal coaching. In addition to MyWW, the company also provides WW for Prediabetes. In one study, volunteers who followed this program significantly lowered their HbA1c level (a long-term measure of blood sugar control) and lost 5.5% of their body weight in six months—and were able to maintain those losses for a year.

Jenny Craig. Established more than 30 years ago, Jenny Craig has about 600 centers around the world. According to a study in *JAMA,* women classified as overweight or obese who followed this program for two years lost 7% of their body weight. Developed by dietitians, the plan relies on a combination of one-on-one personal support from a consultant plus a diet of foods with low energy density. The new Rapid Results program uses a version of intermittent fasting, in which members refrain from eating during a 12-hour "rejuvenation" window, from 7 p.m. to 7 a.m. To get started, members speak with a consultant—in person at a local Jenny Craig center, online via video chat, or by phone—to create an individualized plan.

The program recommends eating three meals and two snacks each day and increasing physical activity as much as possible. Members have the option of preparing their own meals, but the prepared foods have been shown to help people stick with the diet. Close to 100 entrees, snacks, and desserts are available for purchase, and members can supplement these with their own fruits, vegetables, and dairy products. Expected weight loss is about a pound or two a week. Jenny Craig also has a program for people with type 2 diabetes. In one study, adults who started out as overweight or obese lost 9% of their body weight in one year and also lowered their fasting blood sugar and HbA1c.

Meal delivery programs

For people who don't have the time, energy, or interest in cooking, home meal delivery programs can take the guesswork out of weight loss. Rather than providing a meal plan to follow, these programs bring calorie- and portion-controlled meals (and sometimes snacks and desserts) right to your door. Plus, there's no shopping or cleanup. While research on the effectiveness of these services is scant, a small handful of studies hint that they can produce greater weight loss than dieting on your own. Even though these programs can be effective if followed closely, they can be costly.

If you think a meal delivery system would be a good fit for you, consider either of these:

Nutrisystem. Nutrisystem is founded on the concept that eating carbohydrates with a low glycemic index—essentially, carbohydrates that are slowly digested—can help control appetite, hunger, and cravings. Plans are designed for either men or women, with three possible options to choose from: standard, diabetes-focused, or vegetarian. Once weight-loss goals have been achieved, members can choose from three different maintenance plans. All of these can be ordered online or over the telephone and may be customized. Most meals do not need to be refrigerated, making it easy to pack them for work or travel.

Nutrisystem offers three different levels of service: Basic, Uniquely Yours, and Uniquely Yours Ultimate. The latter two include access to weight-loss counselors seven days a week. For times when it's not practical to eat at home, the plan also supplies a guide to dining out, which offers tips for making the best choices at restaurants. Nutrisystem's free NuMi app makes it easy to track food, water intake, and physical activity, and its blog, The Leaf, offers recipes and tips.

BistroMD. This company was developed in 2005 by a physician who noticed that many of her patients struggled to plan and cook healthy meals. Today, it offers more than 150 entrees. Nutritionally, the plan is high in protein and positions itself as being designed to help people who are metabolically prone to gaining weight and resistant to losing it. Calorically, its meals are roughly 40% to 50% lean protein, 20% to 25% healthy fats, and 30% to 35% carbohydrate. Providing a total of 1,100 to 1,400 calories a day, it can be customized to fit the smaller calorie needs of women or the more substantial requirements of men.

Members start by selecting from five program types: standard (women's or men's), gluten-free, diabetes-friendly, heart-healthy, or menopause. Then they choose whether to receive all meals—or just lunches and dinners—for five or seven days. In addition to home-delivered meals, bistroMD offers free virtual support from dietitians and exercise coaches and provides educational emails and newsletters.

Online programs

Thanks to the digital age, diet advice is just a click away. In addition to Web-based options from WW and Jenny Craig, there are an increasing number of diet and exercise programs available online. Most of these programs offer tools that enable you to easily track your eating and exercise habits, count calories, and chart your weight loss. Many also provide meal plans, weight-loss articles, discussion boards, and email advice from experts, including psychologists and registered dietitians. Some feature programs specifically targeted toward men or women, and many offer plans based on popular diets such as low-carb, Mediterranean, or vegetarian.

Do they work? The answer is yes, although not quite as well as face-to-face counseling. The key is engagement. In many studies, the frequency of a user's logins, self-monitoring, chat room attendance, and forum posts correlated with losing weight or keeping it off. If you'd like to give one of these programs a try, here are a few worth considering:

- Atkins (www.atkins.com)
- CalorieKing (www.calorieking.com)
- DASH for Health (www.dashforhealth.com)
- Diet.com (www.diet.com)
- Fooducate (www.fooducate.com)
- Noom (www.noom.com)
- Retrofit (www.retrofitme.com)
- Rise (www.rise.us)
- SparkPeople (www.sparkpeople.com)
- South Beach Diet (www.southbeachdiet.com).

The truth about popular diets

By now you know that there's not one magical diet guaranteed to melt off the pounds. It's also helpful to bear in mind that many diets don't live up to their claims and, in some cases, may even spell trouble for your health. Here's a quick overview of a few popular diet and diet trends. You can find a more in-depth analysis in another Special Health Report from Harvard, *The Diet Review: 39 popular nutrition and weight-loss plans and the science (or lack of science) behind them* (see "Resources," page 53).

Detox diets, cleanses, and juice fasts. Detox diets and cleanses are often laxative concoctions that can cause electrolyte imbalances and dehydration. And they're completely unnecessary. Your body has its own in-house detoxification system: your liver and your kidneys. These two organs work tirelessly to dismantle and remove impurities from your body, so toxins never have the chance to accumulate. As for juice fasts? Vegetable juice can be a good way to bump up

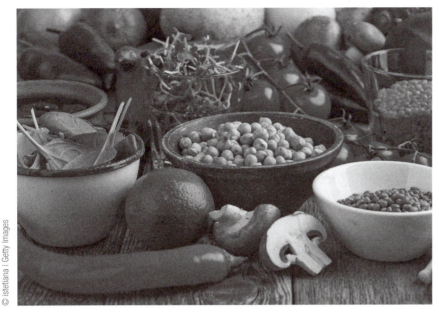

People who follow vegan and vegetarian diets tend to weigh less than nonvegetarians, although it's not clear if this is because of the diet itself or a healthier lifestyle in general.

your produce intake, but it shouldn't be the mainstay of your diet. With a juice diet, you're missing out on fiber, not to mention the protein your body needs to support your liver and kidneys. Since all of these diets are extremely low in calories, they can slow your metabolic rate. Then, as soon as you begin to eat normally again, you're likely to regain the weight that you lost.

Gluten-free diets. Gluten is a protein found in certain grains, such as wheat, barley, and rye. Some people—namely, those with either an autoimmune condition called celiac disease, or with non-celiac gluten/wheat sensitivity—need to eliminate gluten from their diets for medical reasons. A gluten-free diet allows all foods that don't contain gluten, including fruits, vegetables, gluten-free whole grains, meat, poultry, fish, eggs, and dairy. This diet can be very healthful. However, when it comes to weight loss, gluten-free diets provide no advantage whatsoever. What's more, specially formulated gluten-free foods—such as gluten-free breads and pasta—are often high in carbs, refined sugars, and calories.

Intermittent fasting. There are several forms of intermittent fasting, some more extreme than others—such as skipping food every other day. The most robust studies show intermittent fasting does not have a clear weight-loss advantage over simply limiting daily calorie intake. But studies support some metabolic benefits for "time-restricted eating," which limits your daily "eating window." Many people keep their window to eight hours, with an overnight fasting period of 16 hours. For example, if you eat breakfast at 8 a.m., you would not have any food after 4 p.m. a few days per week, or even every day. This practice, especially if breakfast is larger and dinner is smaller, helps synchronize the body's circadian rhythms and promotes metabolic health.

Ketogenic diet. This diet is 75% to 90% fat, 10% to 20% protein, and up to 5% carbohydrates. It forces your body to burn fat instead of glucose (sugar) for fuel. In studies, the keto diet shows some short-term advantage for weight loss and blood sugar management, but there are no long-term studies to offer evidence that people keep the weight off.

Paleo diet. This plan focuses on whole foods such as meat, fish, poultry, eggs, fresh fruits and vegetables, and nuts and seeds, plus coconut, olive, and flaxseed oils. At the same time, it excludes several important food groups, namely grains, legumes, and dairy. As a result, it can lead to deficiencies of calcium and certain B vitamins. It can also be difficult to obtain sufficient fiber on this diet. While a handful of small studies have found that it is effective for short-term weight loss, there is no evidence for long-term results.

Plant-based diets. Even though vegetarians tend to weigh less than nonvegetarians, health experts have had difficulty teasing out whether this is because of their diets or other healthy lifestyle factors. While more research is needed, a small study shed some light on the question. Researchers assigned 63 overweight volunteers to one of five different diets: nonvegetarian, semi-vegetarian (limited in red meat and poultry), pesco-vegetarian (vegetarian with fish), vegetarian (plants plus eggs and dairy), or vegan (plants only). After six months, those who followed the vegan diet achieved the greatest weight-loss success, dropping 7.5% of their body weight, followed by vegetarians, with a 6.3% reduction in body weight. ♥

Weight-loss medications

For many people who aren't able to lose weight with diet and exercise and who are not candidates for weight-loss surgery (see page 45), weight-loss medications (also called anti-obesity drugs) are a viable treatment option. These medications are prescribed by physicians and are usually reserved for people who meet the definition for obesity or those with excess weight plus weight-related health risks, such as heart disease or diabetes. If you have a BMI of 30 or more or a BMI of 27 or more with weight-related health risks and you haven't been able to lose weight through lifestyle changes alone, you may be a candidate.

Because of the tainted history of weight-loss drugs like "fen-phen" (a combination of fenfluramine and phentermine) and over-the-counter products like ephedra (an herbal preparation), misconceptions still exist that these medications are dangerous—or that they are used only for short-term weight loss and aren't effective in the long run. But in combination with lifestyle modification, today's weight-loss drugs provide a long-term treatment option for a great number of individuals with obesity. Most people will lose only a moderate amount of weight with these drugs—about 3% to 9% of body weight on average. However, some people can lose a great deal of weight and maintain their new, lower body weight for years to come—provided that they continue to use the prescribed medication. Stopping the drug almost always brings the weight back.

If you're a candidate for one of these drugs, your physician may prescribe one or more of the recently FDA-approved weight-loss medications, such as liraglutide (Saxenda), naltrexone-bupropion (Contrave), or phentermine-topiramate (Qsymia). For details on these drugs, see Table 7 on page 43.

The history of weight-loss drugs

Only two of today's anti-obesity medications were on the market before 2012: the appetite suppressant phentermine (Adipex-P, Ionamin) and the "fat blocker" orlistat (Xenical). At that time the goal of drug therapy was to reduce appetite or block nutrient absorption. Moreover, when orlistat was developed in the 1990s, the scientific world was focused on the impact of dietary fat on obesity and heart disease. So, at the time it made sense to use a medication like orlistat that would limit the body's ability to absorb fat from food. However, the combination of significant side effects and disappointing results limited the use of orlistat as well as phentermine. Sadly, new drug development was sidelined for years.

That has now changed. As weight-loss experts have gained a better understanding of how the body regulates weight, new drugs have been developed to target the brain as well as gut hormones that influence appetite. Because the brain regulates body weight, it is not surprising that some medications used to treat chronic diseases like depression, seizures, and migraines are also effective in reducing weight. For instance, bupropion, widely known as the antidepressant Wellbutrin, is now a component of the weight-

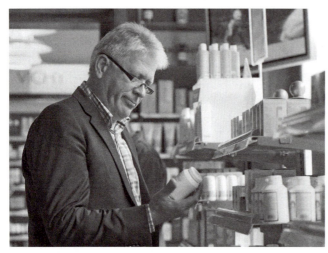

Weight-loss medications may be an option for those with obesity, but over-the-counter supplements that promise to burn fat, curb your appetite, and melt away pounds may be more hype than hope.

loss drug Contrave; topiramate, used to treat seizures and migraines under the name Topamax, is combined with phentermine to make the weight-loss drug Qsymia. In addition to FDA-approved weight-loss medications, your doctor may also prescribe diabetes drugs such as metformin (Fortamet, Glucophage, Glumetza) that can help reduce appetite, block carbohydrate absorption, and reduce sugar production by the liver.

Clinical guidelines suggest that people who respond to a medication (meaning that they lose more than 5% of their body weight) should keep taking that drug to encourage further weight loss. Studies have shown that people who reach this benchmark within the first three months of treatment are more likely to maintain weight loss after a year. Those who do not lose 5% of their body weight within three months should be taken off the medication and be considered for an alternate drug that may be more effective.

In the end, anti-obesity medications may not be a magic bullet, but they can be very effective in helping some people lose weight and keep it off. Because there can be substantial variation in the weight-loss effects—and side effects—it is essential that you don't give up if the first drug you try doesn't work for you. Sometimes you have to try several medications before you find the right one. And, of course, while drug therapy can help you achieve long-term weight loss

Table 7: FDA-approved medications for treating obesity

Here's an overview of the most commonly prescribed weight-loss medications.*

GENERIC NAME (brand name)	HOW IT WORKS	POSSIBLE SIDE EFFECTS	ALSO GOOD TO KNOW
liraglutide (Saxenda)	Mimics a hormone in the gut that sends satiety (fullness) signals to the brain.	Nausea, vomiting, headache, diarrhea, increased heart rate, fatigue.	Also used for diabetes. Given by injection. Should not be used by people with a history or family history of medullary thyroid cancer.
naltrexone and buproprion (Contrave)	Activates brain receptors for dopamine, a brain chemical that helps reduce hunger and impulse eating.	Nausea, vomiting, constipation, diarrhea, dizziness, headache, dry mouth, insomnia, suicidal thoughts.	A combination of an antidepressant and an anti-addiction medication. Should not be used by people with a history of seizures, uncontrolled high blood pressure, bulimia, drug addiction, liver failure, or glaucoma.
orlistat (Alli, Xenical)	Blocks fat absorption in the intestine by up to 30%.	Oily stool leakage, gas, bloating, impaired absorption of fat-soluble vitamins (A, D, E, and K).	Requires supplementation of fat-soluble vitamins and monitoring for vitamin deficiencies. Available over the counter as Alli.
phentermine (Adipex-P, Ionamin, Lomaira)	Suppresses appetite by increasing a brain chemical called norepinephrine that helps reduce appetite.	Dry mouth, constipation, diarrhea, insomnia, headaches, nervousness, restlessness, increased heart rate and blood pressure.	Most commonly prescribed weight-loss medication. Inexpensive. Approved for short-term use (up to 12 weeks). Should not be used by people with a history of heart disease, cardiac arrhythmia, stroke, or uncontrolled high blood pressure.
phentermine and topiramate (Qsymia)	Combination of a stimulant (phentermine) and a medication that decreases cravings and hunger (topiramate).	Increased heart rate, tingling in feet and hands, memory impairment, constipation, dizziness, headaches, fatigue.	Most effective weight-loss medication. Should not be used by people with glaucoma or an overactive thyroid, or who are taking MAOI antidepressants.

*These medications should not be used by women who are pregnant or nursing.

and maintenance, continued focus on a healthy lifestyle and routine monitoring of your weight is also essential for success.

A warning on over-the-counter supplements

A vast array of dietary supplements promise to burn fat, curb your appetite, and help melt away the pounds—all without a prescription. They're typically made from herbs and other natural ingredients, and they're readily available in local stores or via the Internet. But do they work? A 2020 University of Sydney statistical analysis of 54 randomized clinical trials that compared herbal weight-loss medicines to placebos found no evidence to recommend the herbal products. While most of those herbal medicines appeared safe for the short durations of the trials, they largely did not produce clinically meaningful weight loss.

Despite the results of these short-term trials, safety remains a concern. Supplements have been shown to sometimes contain undisclosed prescription drugs—some of which are not approved for use in this country, and many of which have serious, sometimes life-threatening side effects. Case in point: In 2016, a Harvard Medical School study examined 27 performance-enhancing and weight-loss supplements for the presence of oxilofrine, a stimulant that raises heart rate and blood pressure. Even though oxilofrine is banned in the United States, more than 50% of the supplements analyzed contained this substance. Of these, a shocking 43% contained amounts that exceeded the recommended pharmacological dose.

Supplements may also contain toxic ingredients. In 2009, the popular weight-loss aid Hydroxycut was voluntarily withdrawn after the FDA received reports of liver toxicity, seizures, and a type of muscle pain called rhabdomyolysis. Although the current Hydroxycut products no longer contain the troublesome ingredients (notably ephedra), medical literature continues to note adverse effects from the supplement.

Part of the underlying problem is that most popular weight-loss supplements are inadequately tested for safety and effectiveness. Under the Dietary Supplement Health and Education Act of 1994, individual nutrients, herbs, and plants can be sold without such testing, so long as the labeling doesn't make direct health or therapeutic claims. In other words, manufacturers are not permitted to say that their weight-loss aids will cure obesity or make you lose weight, but the law allows them to make more general claims.

Unfortunately, supplement manufacturers routinely base these claims on studies that are much weaker than those used to win FDA approval for prescription drugs. Typically, they include small numbers of people and don't last very long. This has led to a wide array of unfounded assertions on labels and in advertisements. However, the FDA cannot take a product off the market unless it is found to be unsafe. Because the agency can't test every one of the thousands of supplements on store shelves, most face no danger of being removed.

Weight-loss surgery

If you've struggled with your weight and haven't been able to keep excess pounds off with diet and other strategies, including anti-obesity medications, then you may be a candidate for weight-loss surgery (also called bariatric surgery). When used in combination with lifestyle modification, weight-loss surgery has been proven to be the most effective therapy available, yielding long-term results and better health for people with serious weight problems—particularly those who also suffer from weight-related health issues.

Historically, bariatric surgery was believed to cause weight loss by both restricting the amount of food a person is able to eat and also reducing the absorption of calories from the digestive tract into the bloodstream. However, a growing body of research over the last decade has shown that it's not that simple. We are now learning that there are numerous factors responsible for the profound weight loss that occurs after this surgery, including changes in the way you metabolize certain nutrients, variations in your food preferences, alterations in the hormones that control your appetite, and changes in the population of bacteria that live in your digestive tract.

When combined with a healthy lifestyle, the results can be dramatic. Within the first two years after surgery, people typically achieve a maximum weight loss of roughly 20% to 35% of their initial body weight, depending on which procedure they choose. Over time, weight loss tends to decline, but the loss is often maintained in a range that still produces significant health improvements. Diabetes, high blood pressure, high cholesterol, and sleep apnea significantly improve or completely disappear in roughly 60% to 80% of people. These health benefits translate into a nearly 30% lower risk of early death. A 2019 study found that in a group of people diagnosed with both diabetes and obesity, those who had weight-loss surgery significantly lowered their risk of experiencing a heart attack, stroke, heart failure, or similar cardiovascular emergency. Moreover, a range of other health problems also lessen following surgery, including arthritis, asthma, gastroesophageal reflux disease, infertility, sexual dysfunction, and urinary incontinence.

Bypasses, bands, and sleeves

There are three main weight-loss surgical operations—Roux-en-Y gastric bypass, sleeve gastrectomy, and adjustable gastric banding. Of these, the first two operations account for more than 90% of the 196,000 weight-loss surgeries in the United States every year. If you're an appropriate candidate (see Table 8, page 46), you and your surgeon should discuss the various risks and benefits of each technique to decide which surgery is right for you.

Gastric bypass

In Roux-en-Y gastric bypass surgery, the surgeon uses a small portion of the stomach to create a pouch about the size of an egg, which is separated from the rest of the stomach (see Figure 3, page 47). He or she

For people with a BMI of 40 or higher, bariatric surgery may be the surest route to weight loss—and it brings reductions in diabetes and high blood pressure, too. But you must also modify your lifestyle.

Table 8: Are you a candidate for bariatric surgery?

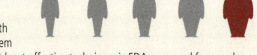

Bariatric surgery may be appropriate for people with a BMI of 40 or higher, along with people with a BMI between 35 and 40 who also have an obesity-related health problem such as diabetes, heart disease, or sleep apnea. Gastric banding, the least invasive but least effective technique, is FDA-approved for people with BMIs of 30 or more who have obesity-related health problems.

To get a rough idea of whether you qualify, find the height that's the closest match for yours; scroll down the column to find your weight; and then scroll to the right to see your weight classification and surgical options. You can also calculate your BMI by going to www.health.harvard.edu/BMI.

HEIGHT	5' 2"	5' 6"	6'	WEIGHT CLASSIFICATION AND SURGICAL OPTIONS
WEIGHT (pounds)	137–163	155–185	184–220	Overweight (25–29 BMI): People in this category generally are not candidates for bariatric surgery.
	164–218	186–247	221–294	Obesity (30–39 BMI): People with a BMI of 35 or over can be candidates if they also have an obesity-related health problem such as diabetes, heart disease, or sleep apnea.
	219 or more	248 or more	295 or more	Severe obesity (40 BMI and over): People in this category may be candidates for bariatric surgery.

then attaches the new stomach pouch to the middle of the small intestine—effectively bypassing the rest of the stomach and the upper part of the small intestine, through which most calories would normally be absorbed. The bypassed part is reconnected farther along the intestine, so digestive fluids continue to drain from the larger section of the stomach. The intestine ends up forming a Y shape—hence, the name Roux-en-Y gastric bypass.

Although the new anatomy cuts down on how much food you are able to eat, this is not the primary reason the procedure results in weight loss. The surgery leads to profound effects on ghrelin (the hunger hormone) and satiety hormones such as GLP-1 and PYY. These changes alter appetite and make you feel full after eating small amounts of food.

The fascinating thing about the changes in these hormones after gastric bypass surgery is that they are the opposite of what occurs after you lose weight with lifestyle modification. For example, after you lose weight via diet and exercise, your level of ghrelin increases, while levels of GLP-1 and PYY fall. That's why you tend to feel hungrier and less full. By contrast, after gastric bypass, ghrelin falls, and satiety hormones rise. Whether this is because food bypasses most of the stomach and a small section of the upper small intestine, or because of other changes that have yet to be discovered, there is something about this surgery that causes the body to respond differently to a lower calorie intake, perhaps making it easier to maintain a lower body weight.

It has been proposed that this surgery changes the body's "set point"—the weight that it wants to maintain. Why? Many of your body's functions, such as blood pressure, blood sugar levels, and hydration, are tightly controlled by your body and brain to maintain balance. For example, if you drink too little, your body will compensate by decreasing the amount of fluid you lose through urine. Similarly, body fat, which is essential for long-term energy storage, is also tightly controlled around a set point. If you eat fewer calories, your body doesn't change your set point. Instead, it responds with changes in hormones that make you hungrier and slow your metabolism. However, it is believed that gastric bypass actually alters the levels of these gut hormones and other physiological parameters, resulting in a set point change. The same is thought to be true of another procedure, sleeve gastrectomy (see page 47).

Gastric bypass usually results in a weight loss of 25% to 35% after one or two years and has shown sustained benefits as long as 20 years later. In addition, it reduces a person's risk for certain chronic diseases, especially diabetes.

Like many other surgical procedures over the past decade, gastric bypass has come to be performed primarily through a laparoscopic approach, which uses tiny instruments inserted into the body through small incisions. This has made the surgery safer, with fewer complications than before, while maintaining effective outcomes.

That said, gastric bypass does have a slightly higher risk of complications than other types of weight-loss surgery. Potential complications include stomach ulcers, stricture (a narrowing of the connection between the stomach pouch and the small intestine), internal hernia (a defect in the abdominal cavity that can trap the intestine), and constipation.

Because the upper part of the small intestine and most of the stomach are bypassed, it's necessary to maintain long-term monitoring of vitamin and mineral levels and lifelong supplementation of vitamin B_1 (thiamine), vitamin B_{12}, calcium, vitamin D, and, for some people, iron.

Sleeve gastrectomy

This operation is now the most commonly performed weight-loss operation in the United States, and it is rapidly growing to be the most common bariatric operation performed worldwide. Like gastric bypass,

Figure 3: The anatomy of weight-loss surgery

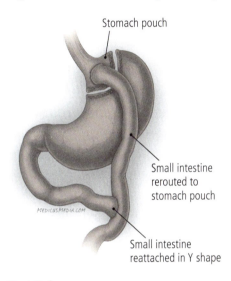
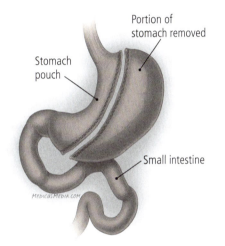
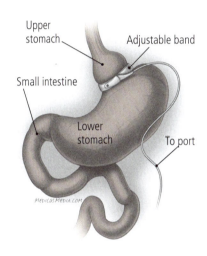

Gastric bypass

Roux-en-Y gastric bypass was developed in the late 1960s after surgeons noticed that overweight patients who underwent a similar gastric procedure designed for stomach ulcers lost weight. A small pouch is created from the upper part of the stomach. The small intestine is cut, and one end is connected to this small stomach pouch. The other end is reattached to the small intestine, creating a Y shape. This allows food to bypass most of the stomach and the upper part of the small intestine, although both continue to produce the gastric juices, enzymes, and other secretions needed for digestion. These drain into the intestine and mix with food at the crook of the Y.

Sleeve gastrectomy

Sleeve gastrectomy was originally used as the first step in weight-loss surgery for people with a BMI of 55 or higher. However, it became a primary weight-loss procedure in 1999. About three-quarters of the stomach is removed to create a narrow banana-sized tube.

An experimental variation, known as endoscopic sleeve gastrectomy (not shown), is under study to see if it may produce similar effects without actually cutting away part of the stomach. Instead, a tube known as an endoscope can be passed down the esophagus and tiny instruments used inside it to make a series of sutures that section off part of the stomach, leaving it with a similar shape to that created in a standard sleeve gastrectomy.

Adjustable gastric banding

A silicone band is placed around the upper stomach to create a small section that has a similar volume to the "pouch" created with gastric bypass. The size of the band can be adjusted by injecting or withdrawing saline through a port implanted just under the skin. The adjustment of the band is used to control hunger and produce a sense of fullness. This procedure has become uncommon because of less favorable long-term results.

it is usually performed laparoscopically, with small instruments inserted through several small incisions in the upper abdomen. It typically results in a weight loss of 20% to 30% of body weight.

In sleeve gastrectomy, the surgeon removes about three-quarters of the stomach, leaving a narrow banana-sized tube (see Figure 3, page 47). Some of the resulting weight loss is thought to be related to decreases in the appetite-stimulating hormone ghrelin, which is primarily secreted from the stomach. In addition, changes in gut hormones may also slow the rate at which food passes through the digestive system, further increasing satiety and promoting weight loss.

One of the advantages of this operation is that it carries a lower risk of complications than gastric bypass surgery. Studies suggest that it's not quite as effective as gastric bypass for weight loss or for improving other weight-related health complications such as diabetes, but it is more effective than gastric banding.

Endoscopic sleeve gastrectomy

Also known as the accordion procedure, this experimental procedure mimics sleeve gastrectomy, but without the need for cutting into the abdomen. Instead, the surgeon inserts an endoscope—a flexible tube with a camera and a suturing device attached—down the patient's throat and into the stomach. The surgeon uses the endoscope to place about 12 sutures in the stomach, leaving it shaped like a tube, as in surgical sleeve gastrectomy.

In the short term, this procedure typically results in less weight loss than standard sleeve gastrectomy, but because the endoscopic procedure is minimally invasive, there may be a lower risk of complications. It's also reversible. Since this procedure is so new, there are no long-term data on how long the weight loss lasts. Unlike gastric bypass and surgical sleeve gastrectomy, endoscopic sleeve gastrectomy is typically done on an outpatient basis.

Gastric banding

This procedure is often called "Lap-Band" surgery, from the trade name of the device placed around the upper stomach to create a small section that is similar in volume to the "pouch" created in gastric bypass surgery (see Figure 3, page 47). Because the gastric band restricts the size of the stomach, it limits the amount of food you can eat. However, unlike gastric bypass or sleeve gastrectomy, it doesn't appear to change hormone levels or have other metabolic effects, making it the least effective of the three procedures. For that reason, as well as a high rate of complications and need for reoperations, gastric banding has fallen sharply in popularity as a surgical intervention for obesity.

Complications are mostly related to the band, which may slip or erode. Another potential complication is dilation of the esophagus, which can occur if the band is too tight; the resulting pressure can cause a pouch to form there, leading to acid reflux, difficulty swallowing, and weight regain.

What to expect after surgery

During the first few months after surgery, your body will adapt to the changes. Regardless of the procedure you have, you will need to be closely monitored by a physician, a dietitian, or both in this early postsurgical phase. Because of the extreme reduction in stomach volume and hormonal changes, your appetite will decrease dramatically, so you'll eat substantially less food. Some people experience vomiting or abdominal pain if they eat too much or too quickly, while others adjust easily. Eating high-carbohydrate meals or snacks may cause sweating, dizziness, nausea, and abdominal cramps—a reaction known as "dumping syndrome" that occurs when a flood of carbohydrates enters the intestine faster than they can be digested. Hydration and daily supplementation (especially of vitamin B_1, vitamin B_{12}, vitamin D, calcium, and, for some, iron) are essential.

The effects of surgery vary among individuals, with potential complications also varying according to the type of operation. The majority of people who undergo weight-loss surgery have few if any complications.

Weight-loss devices

New weight-loss devices have been developed to treat less severe forms of obesity. Although several of these devices have only recently been approved in the United States, some (such as balloons) have been in use in other countries for more than a decade. Currently, these devices are FDA-approved for short-term use in patients with a BMI of 30 to 40 and at least one obesity-associated medical condition.

Intragastric balloons

Gastric balloon systems—such as Orbera and ReShape—produce clinically significant weight loss through multiple mechanisms. In addition to taking up space in the stomach, which has the effect of restricting stomach size, they have been found to increase certain hormones that affect satiety, especially cholecystokinin, which slows down stomach emptying, helping you feel fuller for longer.

Orbera Intragastric Balloon System. Orbera is a grapefruit-sized silicone device that is placed in your stomach and filled with salt solution. It is inserted, uninflated, through your esophagus in a 20- to 30-minute outpatient procedure, so it doesn't require an incision. Because it's resistant to stomach acid, it can remain in the stomach for up to six months. During that period, and after its removal, you work to develop healthier habits that you can later maintain. To this end, you will ideally have regular sessions with a dietitian, fitness trainer, psychologist, and exercise physiologist.

In the United States, Orbera is approved for use for six months along with a supervised diet and exercise program. Although surgeons in other countries report inserting multiple balloons into the stomach—either simultaneously or by a repeat procedure later—this practice is currently not approved by the FDA. Orbera is appropriate only for people who haven't had previous gastric surgery and do not have digestive conditions such as gastritis, ulcers, or hiatal hernia. In addition, people who receive this device are advised to avoid nonsteroidal anti-inflammatory drugs (such as aspirin, ibuprofen, and naproxen) and other stomach irritants during the course of their treatment.

Studies have shown that after six months, people receiving Orbera had lost nearly 7% of their body weight, above and beyond what comparison groups in studies lost by working with the dietitian, fitness trainer, psychologist, and exercise physiologist. Orbera has also been shown to improve diabetes, blood pressure, and cholesterol levels, with relatively few complications. Side effects may include abdominal pain, nausea, and vomiting. However, fewer than 5% of patients require early removal of the balloon. Severe complications, such as bowel obstruction or stomach perforation, are rare, but in the past few years the FDA has received several reports of deaths related to balloon placement. The agency has also received reports of acute pancreatitis and spontaneous hyperinflation (when the balloon suddenly fills with additional liquid or air while in someone's stomach) in users of Orbera and also the ReShape balloon (see below)—conditions that can be life-threatening.

Bear in mind that some people do regain lost weight after the balloon is removed, especially if they fail to maintain the recommended diet and exercise recommendations.

ReShape Integrated Dual Balloon System. ReShape consists of two connected balloons that are inserted into the stomach through a tube placed down the esophagus and then filled with saline. The degree of satiety and resulting weight loss that a person experiences depends on how much space the balloons take up in the stomach. Like Orbera, ReShape is approved for six months along with a supervised diet and exercise program.

Studies have found that people using ReShape lost 7.6% of their initial body weight—versus 3.6% for those given a sham balloon device. They also had improvements in several chronic diseases. Side effects for ReShape are similar to those experienced with Orbera. Similarly, in the past few years, the FDA has received several reports of deaths related to this system.

Other approaches

In addition to balloons, other recently approved devices include a nerve stimulator and a shunt.

The Maestro Rechargeable System. This system, also known as vBloc therapy, uses a pacemaker-like device that is implanted in the stomach. It works by intermittently blocking signals from the vagus nerve. As a result, it slows the rate at which your stomach empties and also helps regulate hunger and satiety signals that are transmitted via the vagus nerve to your brain. However, the precise mechanism of weight loss with the device is unknown. After it is implanted, its settings can be adjusted to maximize its effect.

Clinical trials have demonstrated an average weight loss of 8% with the Maestro system after two years. In addition, it appears to cause few problems, with the most common side effects being heartburn, indigestion, and abdominal pain. Maestro is not appropriate for everyone, though, and is not for use by people with certain conditions, such as liver failure.

The AspireAssist G-Shunt. The AspireAssist G-Shunt helps reduce the number of calories that your body absorbs after a meal by enabling you to remove some of the food in your stomach through a suction tube. The doctor uses an endoscope to place the tube. One end of it is in the stomach. The other end is flush with the skin. Using the tube, you can withdraw approximately 30% of the food from your stomach after a meal and flush it down the toilet. This process takes 10 to 15 minutes to complete.

Studies have shown that people who used aspiration therapy in addition to a diet and exercise program lost more weight after a year compared with people on a diet and exercise program alone. No serious adverse outcomes have been found. However, abdominal pain and infection at the site of the skin port have been noted. People who use AspireAssist seem to eat fewer calories and steer clear of inappropriate eating behaviors or excessive use of the device.

Plenity. Plenity is a pill that releases water-absorbing particles made of cellulose and citric acid into the stomach. Users take three pills with two 8-ounce glasses of water 20 to 30 minutes before lunch and dinner. The particles rapidly absorb the water, expanding to fill about one-fourth of the stomach's capacity, making the user full and less likely to overeat.

Even though Plenity comes in the form of a pill, the FDA classifies it as an "ingested, transient, space-occupying device for weight management and/or weight loss." This is because the particles aren't absorbed into the body; they simply pass through the digestive system and are excreted. A 2018 clinical trial found that people randomly selected to take Plenity lost an average of 6.4% of their body weight in six months, compared with 4.4% of participants who took a placebo pill. Participants who continued to take Plenity beyond six months maintained their weight loss, but did not lose significantly more weight. All study participants were also offered nutritional counseling, instructed to reduce daily food intake by 300 calories, and prescribed daily moderate physical activity.

The FDA approved Plenity in April 2019 for use in people with BMIs between 25 and 40, and as this report went to press, the device was expected to become available in fall 2020. Potential side effects reported in the clinical study include diarrhea, constipation, abdominal pain, and bloating.

Keeping it off

Although weight loss is difficult, keeping the weight off is even harder—and the sad truth is that most people who lose weight will regain it within a few years. However, putting those pounds back on is not inevitable. One in six people classified as overweight or obese is able to maintain a weight loss of 10% of initial body weight for at least one year. This proves that it is indeed possible to keep most of those pounds off, if you know how. And the longer you keep the weight off, the better your chances of sustaining the change over the long run. A small but promising study in the *European Journal of Endocrinology* reported that among people who started out as obese, the longer they could sustain a weight loss, the more likely it was that their bodies would embrace the new weight.

Setting yourself up for success

How can you increase the odds that you'll be in the group of successful dieters who keep the weight off? There are two main strategies.

The first strategy was discussed earlier in this report—exercise. While it is not the most effective approach for losing weight in the first place, it's very important in *maintaining* your new weight. It's an especially effective tool for helping to offset the slowing of metabolism that typically accompanies weight loss. To keep your metabolism revved, the American College of Sports Medicine recommends aiming for more than 250 minutes of moderate aerobic activity each week plus two strength training sessions. (The strength sessions should be at least 48 hours apart to give your muscles time to recover.) Instead of 30 minutes of moderate aerobic exercise five days a week, that means 50 minutes five times a week.

If that seems impossible, try building more activity into your daily activities. Walk or bike to the store rather than hopping in your car. If you take public transportation, get off a few stops earlier and walk. Take stairs, not elevators. Rake leaves instead of using a leaf blower. Try meeting a friend for a walk instead of coffee and donuts. Plan trips and vacations around opportunities to be active, even if it's simply sightseeing on foot. For additional tips, see "Staying motivated," page 34.

At the same time, it's also important to keep focused on what you've learned about healthy eating. We said earlier that you need to find a plan you can stick with in the long run. Well, this is where the long run kicks in. Healthy weight management is not about dieting or counting calories. It's about turning the skills you've learned into habits—eating healthful food that fills you up without loading you down, learning to avoid severe hunger that can send you on a binge, setting up your kitchen so that you don't see tempting snacks, savoring your food so that it provides greater satisfaction, and so forth.

The habits that work for other people will not necessarily work for you. But participants in the National Weight Control Registry—more than 10,000 people who've lost at least 30 pounds and kept the weight off for at least a year—have certain things in common,

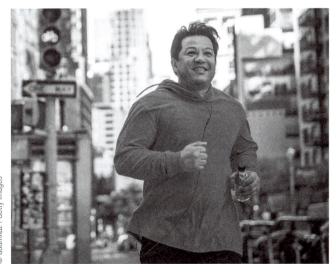

Losing weight is hard, but keeping it off is harder. Exercise is a key factor in maintaining weight loss, in part because it helps keep your metabolism revved instead of letting it dip.

above and beyond the attention they pay to their diets:
- 78% eat breakfast every day.
- 75% weigh themselves at least once a week.
- 62% watch less than 10 hours of TV per week.
- 90% exercise, on average, about one hour per day.

In other words, they maintain an active lifestyle, they keep focused on their weight rather than letting themselves drift off course, and, as mothers so often advise, they eat breakfast.

Maintaining motivation

Of course, to keep up your stellar new habits, you need to maintain your motivation. In the early stages of weight loss, that probably wasn't too difficult. Weight loss was its own reward, as you felt lighter, looked better, and started fitting into smaller-sized clothes. But how do you stay inspired over time—especially when you've hit a plateau where you're no longer losing?

It can be helpful to realize that your body simply isn't programmed to function in weight-loss mode for a prolonged period of time. Eventually everyone's weight loss slows down and levels off. This isn't because your weight-loss plan isn't working. Rather, it's because your body has adapted by reducing your metabolism to support the decreased energy needs of your newer, smaller body size—so it's actually an achievement.

During periods of maintenance or plateaus, you may find that your brain is making you feel more hungry in an attempt to force you to regain the weight you've lost. As a result, you may have more cravings and feel less full. Keep in mind that this body-brain tug-of-war is to be expected, and it's likely going to be your biggest challenge.

Studies show that the six- to 12-month mark is a pivotal juncture where most people hit a plateau and begin to regain some of their lost weight. You should anticipate this and understand that it is not a sign of failure and that it's natural to regain some of those lost pounds over time. During this time, staying the course and focusing on your health should be your primary goals.

When your resolve starts to weaken, these strategies can help:
- Make a list of the reasons why you want to maintain your weight loss—perhaps you found out you were at risk for a serious illness or you just feel better when you weigh less. Put your list in a place where you will see it every day.
- In addition, write yourself a letter, outlining your reasons for wanting to lose weight and your sense of achievement at having come this far. Tuck it into an envelope and put it in your desk or dresser drawer. If you feel yourself backsliding, pull it out and reread it, to remind yourself that weight loss is doable—after all, you've done it already.
- Post "before" and "after" pictures on your refrigerator as a reminder of how much better you look and feel having taken off some weight.
- Give yourself a nonfood reward for successfully maintaining your new habits—for example, a new bestseller or tickets to a show you've been wanting to see.
- Recruit a supportive—but not bossy—friend or family member to help keep you on track. This will make you feel accountable.
- Have a plan for situations where you are offered tempting food. Script possible responses for politely but firmly declining food you didn't plan for, and practice them before you actually need to use them.
- Actively seek out friends who are interested in healthy cooking and eating, or who enjoy being physically active.
- Try not to beat yourself up if you splurge or give into temptation. It happens. Just pick yourself up, move on, and resolve to do better next time.
- Learn from your lapses. Lapses are so normal, experts actually consider them to be part of the process of establishing new habits, so acknowledge your lapses with self-compassion, then brainstorm some solutions. For example, if your downfall is snacking at night, try closing the kitchen after dinner. If you've eaten three good meals and two snacks during the day, you shouldn't need more snacks at night.

Finally, realize that it's not always about your conscious decisions. Weight loss is more about how your body is responding to a certain diet, exercise routine, or sleep cycle. So stop thinking in terms of "success" and "failure," and always keep in mind that weight loss—and maintenance—are part of a dynamic ongoing cycle that requires a lifetime of healthy habits. ▼